Know Yourself

*and you will be able to atune your whole being to
the positive rhythms of life. It's not magic, and you
don't need to enroll in some expensive course or
spend long years at a guru's feet. The key to your
future good health and success in life lies in your
own subconscious mind, in the type of meditative
thinking that produces the slow Alpha-wave cycles
in your brain and enables you to channel your mind
and body into positive, creative, healing patterns.*

Now, best-selling author Jess Stearn provides you
with the complete instructions he himself followed
in learning to "think Alpha," and offers his own
experiences with both Alpha-Thinking and Biofeedback, as well as those of a number of his fellow
students, as proof of what the strength of your own
mind can do. And you, too, have the tools to establish contact with yourself and develop your total
being. All it takes is your own desire and—

THE POWER OF ALPHA-THINKING

SIGNET Books of Interest

The Power of Alpha-Thinking —Miracle of the Mind

by JESS STEARN

With an Introduction by
Dr. John Balog

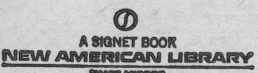

A SIGNET BOOK
NEW AMERICAN LIBRARY
TIMES MIRROR

Foreword

I have written this book with the hope that others will join in exploring the hidden powers of the mind. After four years of research, carefully documenting so many wonders, I am still amazed by the infinite potential of the subconscious. For the person wishing to develop these new dimensions, I have relived the program that introduced me to this world of tomorrow, with its promise of self-fulfillment on a plane never before conceived by man. Someday soon we may all recognize that whatever the human mind can visualize it can achieve with knowledge and faith. The world of inner space begins with the individual and ends with him. He is his own guide and his own healer. He can make himself ill or well. He can be happy or bored, resentful or exalted, productive or stagnant. With the miracle of subconscious meditation and visualization, he has the tools to establish contact with himself at his deepest level and develop an inner awareness and calm that make the boundless universe his unspoken ally. For the first time, in achieving self-mastery, he may know what it is to become truly the master of his fate and the captain of his soul.—J.S.

Contents

An Introduction

by John Balog, M.D.

The new powers of the mind explored in this book presage one of the most hopeful trends of the century. The union of Western technology and ancient meditative practices may yet lead us out of the Age of Anxiety with its increasing abuse of tranquilizing drugs and the growth of psychosomatic disorders. In the past, when a doctor told someone, "It's all in your head," little could usually be done for the patient in any predictably effective way. But now, with varying thought controls, we have come upon a method of getting it out of the head.

I can foresee Biofeedback visualization and meditation continuing to develop in many useful directions. As it is, we are now able to teach the average person to school his own muscle response, regulate his blood flow, and manipulate his own brainwaves to his own singular advantage. With this new awareness, we can "see" ourselves clearly and readily influence our own behavior, applying this technique to a variety of ailments, from gastrointestinal problems and tension headaches to regaining muscle control after becoming paralyzed.

It is important to recognize that brainwaves, as measured by the EEG, have been correlated with certain experiences and convenient designations that have been applied to certain frequency ranges. The first rhythmical frequency to be observed on the EEG was eight to thirteen cycles per second. It was described by the German physician Berger, and called the Alpha wave because it was the first to be discovered. Considerable interest is now shown because this pattern is associated with calm, alert, pleasant, as well as meditative and introspective experiences. The Alpha wave was initially observed in the occipital or posterior brain, which is usually associated with vision. But Alpha waves have also been observed at other surface locations of the brain. For practical purposes we might say that Alpha is the border line between conscious and subconscious activity. Problem-solving conscious activity is usually associated with fast, low-voltage brainwaves commonly called Beta waves. These range from thirteen cycles per second to as high as forty cycles. The slower, high-voltage brainwave patterns, known as Delta and Theta, are associated with subconscious activity and are often mingled with the Alpha, which is associated with creativity, dreams, and sleep. Brilliant discoveries have been reported in this state by scientists and inventors who appeared to be dozing. In training for the Alpha-Theta state, students seek to achieve the same level of creativity that these men attained inadvertently. Since all this is so new, and some few are overly suggestible, students in Biofeedback training and in the so-called Alpha courses should carefully check the qualifications of their teachers and be assured that they have a record of responsibility over an extended period. The experience itself should be measured along with the result.

In Biofeedback, of course, we have a more explicit way of measuring results than in the average commercial Alpha course. We have been able to effectively correlate Biofeedback training with specific instances of self-help.

Changes in muscle tension and hand temperature, even without the Biofeedback machines, are something we can immediately sense. However, brainwaves, by their hidden nature, appear to be mysterious and ephemeral. But these can be measured as well, and consequently modified, when electroencephalograph (EEG) electrodes are placed on the scalp and attached to an amplifier, meter, or lights. In this training to deliberately produce Alpha and Theta brainwaves, many have already been helped, not only with their ailments but in the areas of solving problems and improving creativity. Biofeedback has also become a useful tool in psychotherapy.

At times, a combination of the three Biofeedback devices has been used to help people with insomnia, epilepsy, cardiac arrythmias, chronic pain, bladder control, bruxism (grinding of the teeth), premature ejaculation, hypertension, and a host of other conditions.

But the ultimate, I believe, is yet to come, as the public

program develops and grows. I can picture the widespread use of Biofeedback training in the schools, as part of the regular curriculum in health education. Children can then beneficially experience altered states of consciousness without recourse to the hazardous side effects of alcohol and drugs, so often associated with so-called mystical or mind-expanding experiences. As the multitudes achieve voluntary control over mind and body, I can foresee a resulting decrease in stress-related illnesses and a widespread improvement in general well-being, with a resulting drop-off in medications.

I also hopefully foresee a revolutionary miniaturization of the Biofeedback equipment now in use, so that the average person will be able to get his own feedback about his internal states outside of the doctor's office. Already we have a temperature device to be worn like a wristwatch, and a portable muscle responder, making an audible sound as tension rises. This could be used even when driving, without having to take the eyes off the road.

The EEG (brainwave measuring machine) readily lends itself to portable units, which can be used at home. In time, an indwelling catheter in the vein may also measure blood sugar response for diabetics or cholesterol for those on low-fat diets, as well as be a measure of stress. Finally we might develop devices to monitor cell growth, and through our own mind power, control cancerous tumors.

Working with author Jess Stearn in this pioneering field has been a stimulating experience. His own exploration of the new frontiers of the mind, so that others can follow in his footsteps, is certainly a valuable and unique contribution. Read on and marvel at the hidden powers of the mind—which could just as easily be your mind as well.

Chapter 1

The Unbelievable Mind

"You were able to correctly diagnose an illness, not knowing or seeing that person?"

Twenty-three-year-old Cathy Francis nodded her head. "I was given only that person's age and sex."

I looked at my young visitor as if she were out of her mind. It didn't faze her in the least.

"I closed my eyes and saw the cancer clearly. It was lodged in the woman's stomach, and I recognized it as cancer, even though I had never seen a cancer before."

"How would you know it was cancer?"

"The word stood out in my mind as clearly as the cancer itself. It was a large, forbidding mass."

She shuddered.

We had been discussing the hidden potential of the mind, in a general way, when she made her startling claim.

"Even Edgar Cayce," I observed, referring to the greatest of American mystics, "required a subject's name and address, plus a request for help, before he went into trance and diagnosed illnesses at a distance."

"Nevertheless," she said firmly, "it happened just as I said."

She looked hardly old enough to be out of high school, not to mention college.

"What would you be doing with cancer?"

"That was only incidental." She gave me a disarming smile. "You could do as much yourself, if you took the course I did."

"I have no desire to impersonate a doctor."

She shook her head. "That was only an example of inner awareness, of my subconscious mind. They call it going into your levels. It has nothing to do with medicine. I could have tuned into a tree, a mountain, or a dog."

I looked out on the surf lapping at my doorstep, momentarily reassured by its reality, and wondered if this aspiring young actress was putting me on because of my interest in the metaphysical field.

"Where was this woman when you read for her?"

"Presumably at home."

"How did you know about her?"

"Another member of the class proposed her as a subject."

"Was she aware of your interest?"

"Not that I know of. Her case was given to me in class to show my progress in developing Alpha brainwaves."

It sounded like so much mumbo-jumbo.

"And why should being in Alpha make you psychic or broaden the dimensions of your mind?"

"Why not find out for yourself? No matter what I tell you, you won't accept it, just as I wouldn't before I went through the experience."

"How long does it take to develop the kind of Alpha-thinking that enables you to see inside stomachs?"

She laughed. "The course takes four days, about forty hours in all."

"You could do this in four days?"

"Others did more."

It all seemed so bizarre. And even if true, what was it but some psychic trick that didn't serve any useful purpose?

She looked at me in surprise. "I thought I had made it clear that essentially this is a problem-solving device, designed to make you so super-aware that you know all about your hangups, and your friends' as well."

In our case, it apparently hadn't solved the problem of communication. "What are some problems that Alpha-thinking clears up?"

"It has helped people with weight control, reducing with incredible ease. Others have learned to sleep at will, ease tension, get rid of severe headaches, speed-read, and improve their memories."

"Do they walk on water?"

She sighed. "I told you that you would have to find out for yourself.

And so began an experience which altered my life in

more different ways than even Yoga had years before. It was to be a mind-opening, eye-boggling adventure, fraught with skepticism and misgivings, yet opening up eventually onto a broad vista of the human potential as boundless as the universe itself.

I was not aware of any of this, of course, as I faced a pleasant-featured Alexander Everett across the table in suburban San Rafael. Months before, the handsome, middle-aged Englishman had settled in San Francisco and welded together a mind-training organization. He was apparently well-qualified. He had founded a boys' school in England, at Henley-on-Thames, later teaching in Texas. He had worked with José Silva, the pioneer of commercial mind control in this country, who had learned about the Alpha technique from an Army psychiatrist, then experimented with imaginative Alpha-prone children before launching his own awareness program.

Everett likewise specialized in self-awareness with the supersensitive subconscious mind arbitrarily assigned to the slower Alpha and Theta brainwave cycles, usually appearing together, and Beta brainwaves, the most common, reflected in normal usage of the five senses. Delta, seldom encountered normally, was a deep, trance-like state.

"Talking together, sizing each other up," said Alexander, "we are in Beta, and see each other as we seem to be. If we delved into the deeper layers of our mind, into our Alpha levels, we would see each other as we really are."

Everett readily recalled Cathy Francis. "She was the average student," he said, "nothing spectacular."

"You don't think it unusual," I said, "for a girl to close her eyes and correctly diagnose a cancer case miles away?"

"It's a matter of tuning into the right frequency," he answered nonchalantly, "just as you would a radio. Anything any man-made machine does, man should be able to do."

It seemed reasonable, but hardly practical. In 1910, Germany's Dr. Johannes Schultz had introduced autogenic mind-training, with its potential for solving psychosomatic problems, and the world had shrugged its shoulders and looked away. And yet Alexander Everett had structured a successful business out of it.

"You are selling this course," I said, "and making money out of it."

He was not in the least defensive. "There's nothing wrong about charging for something, as long as the person's getting his money's worth. Essentially we want to make this a better world. People of different faiths and nationalities are just going to have to learn to get along with one another, or the human race will become extinct."

And what did brainwaves have to do with international compatibility?

"If you have no feeling for your neighbor, how can you have it for strangers and foreigners? With the subconscious mind, you see things more clearly, and one of the things you see is that we have to love to survive. You can't love anyone else unless you love yourself. The world is fouled up because so many people hate themselves and take it out on others."

"So how do you learn to like yourself?"

"By going within and finding out who you are, at the subconscious state. The deeper you go within, through meditation and visualization, the more likely you are to find the perfect self within, beautiful, loving, and unafraid."

As we sat together in his office, watching the traffic outside, I still had no sense of reality. It was all words.

He smiled reassuringly. "We're having a study group tonight in a teacher's home. Stop by and see how it works. Our graduates get together, usually once a week, to discuss their progress and to work out specific problems—personal hangups like being too fat, inability to concentrate, smoking, insomnia, nervousness, frustration, headaches, high blood pressure, and other illnesses, usually of a psychosomatic nature."

As he talked, he occasionally plucked a grape from a bowl. "I'm dieting," he explained.

"Why not program yourself with Alpha?"

He carefully selected another grape. "I did; that's why I'm lunching on grapes."

"Couldn't you just think yourself thin?"

He frowned. "Let me see how I can put this so you

have an idea of what we are trying to accomplish. The average person works at ten percent of potential. That's all your conscious Beta mind can do for you. But the mind has many dimensions, and the untouched potential lies at a deeper level than we ordinarily use. It is even located in a different hemisphere of the brain, and is sometimes called the 'old brain' because it is the rudimentary brain which animals also possess.

"To contact this instinctual side of the mind, mind students enter an altered state of awareness. They relax body and mind, blocking out sensory impulses, and concentrate on visualizing, .to develop the subconscious pattern that makes the individual super-aware.

"After blocking out the rational, intellectual mind, the student slips into the deeper levels of his mind and creates an imaginary workshop, decorates and furnishes it in his mind so that he can feel comfortable and productive there. He puts in an imaginary screen, similar to a motion picture screen, and it is on this Screen of the Mind that he floats the problems he intends to solve. Always keep in mind when you go into these levels that you become more loving and kind, have a greater depth of understanding, and gain more rapport with your family, friends, and those with whom you work. With this dagger of his mind, the student can tune into almost anybody or anything he puts on this Screen."

I still had no idea how ordinary people were transformed into psychic marvels. "How can he visualize somebody he doesn't even know?"

"But he does know what they're like, for he gets onto their wave length with his subconscious mind."

"And he becomes a receiver in four days?"

"He becomes aware," Alexander corrected, "of his capacity for reception in these four days. And with practice, he gains psychic awareness: the power to heal, create, and to communicate effectively with people he never understood before."

This miracle of the mind began with self-knowledge. "I hate to keep saying this, but you really have to experience mind-training to understand how it works."

I recognized the subconscious force, but thought of it as given only to the few. I had seen the Reverend Douglas

Johnson of Los Angeles heal the ill, felt the heat from his hands over an ailing body. The Swami Rama, tested at Menninger Clinic, in Topeka, Kansas, lowered his heartbeat to twelve beats a minute, then stopped the flow of blood from his heart, to demonstrate the subconscious mind's remarkable control of the body.

Now I was told that many could do what seemed unbelievable when done by only the few.

I looked forward to the study group.

About fifty people were sprawled around the San Rafael living room. They were mostly in their twenties, though I did notice every age bracket, including a handful of children. I settled myself next to an attractive young woman with azure blue eyes. She was closely watching a man introduced as an instructor. He was tall and dark, handsome in a rather sleek way, and he spoke with a glib assurance that tripped off warning bells.

"If you have any kind of a problem, or are concerned over somebody else's problem," he announced, "merely give me the person's age and sex, and I will tune into that person and surround him with light."

The young woman hesitated, then raised her hand.

The instructor boldly appraised her. "Yes?" His voice held just the right note of professional inquiry.

She spoke up in a musical voice. "I have in mind a seventeen-year-old girl."

"All right." He smacked his hands together. "We'll examine the problem." He closed his eyes, and his steepled hands began to weave slowly downward from his head. "You are concerned about this girl," he said with an acuteness less than startling.

His hands had now dropped below the chin. "This girl has a problem with her throat, but it will respond to proper treatment."

His eyes were still closed. "I get a connection between you and this girl. She is related, your sister." He hesitated. "She ran away from home, and you are concerned about her whereabouts."

The youthful beauty's face was set in noncommittal lines.

His hands continued downward. "I see a darkness in the stomach area. She should see a doctor."

He opened his eyes and stared challengingly across the room.

"Thank you," she said softly.

I drew my head close to hers.

"How about it?" I whispered.

She grimaced. "He was wrong on everything except my concern."

I took stock of her once again. "So you don't believe?"

"Oh yes, I do. He just didn't do the job. He was trying to make an impression."

I took her aside. "Is the girl your sister?"

She made a surprising reply. "No, my daughter."

"Your daughter! You don't look more than twenty-five yourself."

"I'm thirty-four," she said simply.

I made an educated guess. "Your daughter has a drug problem?"

"Whose daughter hasn't?" she answered a little wearily.

"And a problem with a young man?"

Her lips parted in the hint of a smile. "You're guessing, but you're still an improvement."

"Well, what is the problem?"

She sighed. "My daughter is married to a violent young man, who is destroying her spirit by beating her every time she tries to express her independence."

"Such as leaving him?" I said.

"Right."

I waved an arm. "So why believe in any of this?"

"I have seen it work, and did it myself while taking the course."

"Then why not try it yourself?"

"I didn't like what I saw. I was hoping for somebody less involved to tell me something different."

I glanced around the room at little clusters of people weaving their hands over their cases and was planning my exit when I heard my name above the noise.

At the far end of the room, a tall young man with sandy hair stopped weaving his hands long enough to catch my eye.

His voice carried across the room. "You have been observing all this activity without really knowing whether

7

the information is correct. I would like to demonstrate one case for you alone."

"Why me?" I asked in surprise.

He was refreshingly candid. "We would like you to write about the Alpha as you did about Yoga and Edgar Cayce, and let people know that Alpha-thinking can help them."

He had the room's attention.

"And how will you do this?"

"Give me the age and sex of anybody you know with a problem, and I will tune in."

"No name or address?"

"That will be enough."

"Are you a psychic?"

He smiled. "I'm an accountant."

We chatted for a few moments. John Burnham was twenty-eight and worked in San Francisco. He had taken the Alpha course but a few weeks before, and it had already changed his life.

"What did it do for you specifically?" I inquired.

"There was a ten-thousand-dollar discrepancy in our accounts, and even the computer couldn't locate it. So I dropped down into my Alpha levels and visualized the computer at work, and picked up the computer error."

"I trust you were properly rewarded."

"They gave me a raise. I knew exactly what it would be."

I went over in my mind the people I knew with problems. The list seemed endless.

He stood waiting politely. "Be sure," he stressed, "that it is somebody with a tangible problem."

"Why is that?" I asked.

"There should be a motivation for help, idealistically, and it should be verifiable."

"All right," I said finally, "a twenty-four-year-old girl."

By this time, I had drawn closer to the steps on which he stood, a little above the crowd.

He pushed back a strand of hair, then closed his eyes. A serene expression came over his face. His hands began their weaving course downward, as if he were balancing on a tightrope.

"Why," I asked, "do you keep moving your hands?"

"We are better able to visualize the body this way."

His hands were at his shoulders. "This girl is tall and beautiful, with a glowing complexion."

"That could apply to many people," I said.

He shook his head. "No comments are necessary."

"Do you see anything?"

Eyes closed, he waved me off.

The thirty-four-year-old girl at my side, almost forgotten in this diversion, whispered, "You're interrupting his concentration."

At the waist, his hands hesitated, dropped two or three inches, then stopped.

"This girl," he said slowly, "has a problem in the pelvic cavity. I see a darkness, an infection. It has had a debilitating effect."

He opened his eyes and looked at me inquiringly.

"Very interesting," I said. "She does have something wrong there, after having a child, and nobody seems able to help."

He seemed reassured.

"Can you pick out the problem?" I asked.

He shrugged. "I'm not a doctor, and so can't consciously interpret what I see."

"Nevertheless," I said, "you have done very well."

I was about to turn away when he held up his hand. "If that was all, it would be little more than a parlor trick."

I stopped short. "What more is there?"

"We must help this girl. That's what it's all about."

"How do you do that?"

He peered over my head into the room. "I am going to ask the graduates and instructors to go down into their Workshops, put this girl on their imaginary Screens, and throw a protective light around her."

He turned back to me. "We are going into our subconscious levels and concentrate, so that she will change her doctor and get the proper treatment."

I was intrigued by this rather bizarre turn. Perhaps a dozen people had closed their eyes and appeared to be meditating, palms up. The beautiful girl with the azure eyes was sitting against the wall, Yoga-fashion, her lids shut and a look of angelic serenity on her face.

Many youthful lips were moving, as if in prayer. Where, I asked myself, was this help coming from, and how was it to materialize? Even if they produced some form of radiating energy, how did they direct it properly? It was truly incredible.

The meditation came to an end, and John Burnham sauntered over.

He smiled easily. "I hope we were able to help that girl."

"How," I asked, "does a simple accountant become a genius overnight?"

"Anybody can do what I did," he said modestly. "All he needs to do is get into Alpha or Theta, the Alpha or Alpha-Theta state, tune into the universe around him, and get it working for him. There's nothing mysterious about it, once you understand that there is something of the infinity of the universe in all of us and that we all are connected through our connection to the whole."

I had about all I could handle in a weekend. I was glad to get back to Southern California and think it over, alone. If it was true, as John Burnham said, that he had altered his life by adding a new dimension of the mind, then anybody could do it—the millions suffering from frustration, malaise, depression, and others with little purpose save that of putting one day after another. If some natural law—God's law—could be invoked to assist some nameless girl in some nameless place, then it could be mustered for anybody.

Two days later I telephoned the twenty-four-year-old girl who had been the subject of the demonstration. "Don't nag," she said quickly. "I made an appointment yesterday with my mother's doctor, and I hope everybody is satisfied."

Two weeks later, with new treatment, Kathy Bleser was perfectly well. There had been no psychic healing, nothing mysterious or occultish, merely a routine changing of physicians. Without Burnham's demonstration, I would have thought no more about it. Even so, how could the thoughts of strangers influence the action of a person they had never heard of?

How intriguing—the idea that somebody could sink into his levels and put himself into somebody else's head, or put that person's head on! I could imagine all kinds of possibilities. Could I project, say, into the President's head and advise him on foreign and domestic policy? If John Burnham could influence somebody he didn't know, why couldn't I climb into my publisher's mind and influence the books I believed in? Was there any reason why I or anybody else in these inner levels couldn't persuade an indifferent lady to return his affection?

"With mind development," Alexander assured me, "you can influence anybody you like, as long as the intention is good."

Alpha was a force for good, not evil, if Everett was correct in his assumption that the inner core of man is incorruptible.

I saw ample evidences of this new mind power in everyday relationships between husband and wife, mother and child, employer and employee, salesman and client, doctor and patient. Children could be Alpha-trained more easily than adults because, less logically oriented, they were so often in the imaginative Alpha state anyway. And women more easily than men, since they so frequently called on their intuition in dealing with the rational, physically dominant male.

"It is only a question of getting into the proper frequency," explained Charlene Afremow, a San Rafael housewife and mother, and Alexander's resident instructor. "It works something like a radio, once you're in your levels. You turn the dial, and you get a station on one frequency; move it a little more, and you have still another frequency, with a new station coming in equally clear."

What the radio could do, the schooled mind could do even better. Charlene had put her whole family into mind-training, to smooth out the wrinkles of family togetherness. "For mutual understanding, it was as important for my growing son to know me as for me to know him." And so the boy took the course as well. Their relationship was by no means unique in a world of changing values. "Twelve-year-old George and I had reached the usual impasse of working mothers and subteeners who feel neglected. We would retreat into ourselves, finding it difficult to discuss the problems we were creating for each other. I went into my levels and got into George's head, and realized that he wasn't just being inconsiderate, but was expressing the hurt deep down because he didn't think I cared enough for him. Loving him, it was inconceivable to me on a conscious level that he could think this."

After taking his mother's course, George dipped deep into her subconscious and saw clearly a mother's hopes and aspirations, still unexpressed in her conscious thinking. Never again did he doubt her love.

"As we all should know," observed Charlene, "love is the food that children grow on. It makes them straight and tall and self-reliant, and that's what I now saw happening to George."

Suppose George had not taken the course?

She could only shrug. "Then he wouldn't have seen any more than any twelve-year-old boy."

I had a glimpse of George's new perception.

I had gone from the Afremow home in San Rafael to nearby Sausalito to visit a friendly tycoon aboard his hundred-foot cruiser. He was sitting with a marine engineer, discussing a leak which had kept the ship in port.

He looked up as I arrived. "We just got it repaired," he said, "and now I can take that cruise."

"It beats all," said the engineer, "how you located that leak."

The millionaire smiled mysteriously. "I have my ways." His eyes followed the engineer down the gangplank.

"What was that all about?" I asked.

He laughed uproariously and slapped his thigh in jubilation. "I've had engineers crawling over this place looking for the leak, without any success. It looked like we might have to start tearing into the boat." He laughed again, hardly able to contain himself. "Lots of people heard of my dilemma, and the next thing I knew young George Afremow was asking me if he could help, and I told him I could use all the help I could get."

"And?" I coaxed him along.

"And so he went down into his levels, put his thinking cap on, and saw the leak as big as life. It was just where he said it was."

My jaw must have dropped, for the millionaire grinned. "I was amazed, but grateful." He waved an arm toward the dock. "Of course, I didn't tell the engineers where the help came from. They would have thought I was off my rocker."

He estimated that George had saved him as much as ten thousand dollars. "He's a good man to have around."

I asked George about his feat the next time I saw him.

He blushed modestly. "I just saw it all in my Workshop."

"How did you happen to do it?"

He looked at me shyly. "I wanted to help the owner of the boat," he said. "He helps lots of people, and I like him for that."

The wonders of Alpha never ceased—apparently.

Chapter 2

Miracles or Mirage

Even with all of Alexander's postulations, I was still rather confused as to how the subconscious mind—the Alpha and Theta particularly—express themselves beneficially.

I had been told that the subconscious mind had ten times the power of the conscious mind, enabling ninety-pound weaklings to perform feats of strength in the Alpha-Theta state, but I still had no idea, functionally, what made this transformation possible.

"So you slow up your thought processes," I said to the gray-haired authority on hypnosis and mind-expansion, "and it all begins to happen magically."

"Not magically at all," said Dr. Jules Bernhardt, of Los Angeles' San Fernando Valley. "There's a very definite physical process taking place. I tell my students that the subconscious doesn't know the difference between the real and the imaginary. The subconscious has no sense of humor. It is very literal and accepts what it is told in the way of visualization and meditation. The important thing in improving ourselves, in becoming more aware, is not movement but change, and this is accomplished not through conscious will power, but by educating our imaginations to make the choices that help."

The body, and the conscious mind as well, almost immediately respond to the pattern established in the Alpha-Theta state.

"Once we accept the visualized suggestion, the automatic nervous system experiences it, and the desired changes toward calm and peace of mind suddenly take place. The nerve ends, which may have been previously disassociated, come together in a coordinated synapse or juncture of the dendrites and axones. Every time we visually experience a coordinated bodily process, these nerve ends come closer together, until the nervous system is working smoothly and effortlessly, without strain."

Other changes take place as well, and it is all self-initiated. "We are responsible for our thoughts, and our thoughts are responsible for bodily changes, even to influencing the blood sugar, the circulation, the metabolism, respiration and any other automatic function, since the mind, functioning on this Alpha level, is given a will of its own in the struggle for survival."

At all times there is an appeal to strengths, not weaknesses. Still, there had to be some acknowledgment by the intellectual mind that it could no longer handle things before the subconscious mind could be invoked and programmed positively.

Bernhardt had it all worked out in simple terms. "The subconscious, which does creative problem-solving, solves the self-help problem after the Beta mind has gone into Alpha-Theta and asked for assistance, saying, in effect, 'I don't know what to do any more, will you help me?'"

Bernhardt tells his students at his North Hollywood institute that changes, to be beneficial, have to be psychological, physiological and philosophical, all readily possible through controlling the brainwaves. "To create, go into Alpha in a state of relaxed concentration; Theta, if you want to dream helpfully, for you can't live without dreams, which are the other side of the mind, and into Delta to sleep at a level renewing the vital forces."

As Alpha-Theta opens up new pathways in the nervous system, there is consequent improvement in mental attitudes, physical faculties and nervous integrity, meaning the nervous system becomes more stable and reliable.

If all this was true, I wondered why everybody didn't profit from it.

Bernhardt had been observing patients and students for thirty years. "Not everybody"—he smiled—"wants to survive. Emerson once said, 'Be careful of what you wish for, or you may get it.'"

Bernhardt, like Everett, maintained that the feeling

of love was paramount in building a self-image to bring the individual the desired calm and creativity.

"You have to love yourself properly, and not see yourself as unworthy, to touch your life and that of others with your special uniqueness."

Loving was where the transformation for good lay. And it was done with imagery, with the creativity of Alpha. For as the great Indian master, Sai Baba, had said, "There is only one Yoga discipline that matters—not the Hatha Yoga of the conditioned body, or the Raja Yoga of the orderly mind, but the Prem Yoga—Prem meaning the highest aspect of love, loving the Divine Self, the God Self."

Relaxation, self-improvement and healing somehow seemed all interwoven. But there still had to be a sense of expectancy if anything was to come of the relaxed concentration that appeared to be a prelude to beneficial change. "Otherwise," said Bernhardt, "it is merely a game."

Every teacher, of course, was a former student, and diligently practiced his meditations so as to at least keep abreast of his class. With constant repetition, as Bernhardt pointed out, the nervous system could now serenely establish a pattern of subconscious behavior capable of achieving apparent miracles. For the most part, the miracle-workers were modest people who only confirmed what had been said by the wisest teacher of all two thousand years ago: "Ask, and you will receive; seek, and you will find; knock, and the door will be opened."

Into that open door anybody with a wish for survival could take a giant step and hopefully move forward. Some of the presumed miracles were so incredible that they required all the validation that they evidently had. It could happen to anybody at any time, if the transmitter and receiver were in harmony. Yet I was still skeptical when one of Alexander Everett's former teachers, Dorothy Nelson of the Sanjaya Center in West Los Angeles, called one day to say she had a rare testimonial. "It is so remarkable a cure," said she, "that I can hardly believe it myself."

Quite simply, if the information was correct, she had wrought a miracle. The subject was a sixty-nine-year-old woman who had developed cataracts in both eyes. Hazel Wightt was a widow, and she lived in the Brentwood section of Los Angeles. She had been examined by her ophthalmologist of thirty-five years, and he had prescribed not bifocals, but trifocals, glasses with three ranges of vision, until the cataracts had ripened to the point where they could be surgically removed.

She had not yet received the glasses and had been stumbling about in broad daylight, unable to read or write. She had worked as a bookkeeper to augment her widow's pension, but gave up the job when the figures became a hopeless blur.

In church on a Sunday, she had tearfully related her problem to an old friend, who was familiar with the work done in meditation by Dorothy Nelson and her graduates.

"Are you sure," the friend asked, "that you have cataracts?"

She dried her tears. "There is no question of it."

He had looked at her speculatively. "Do you believe that Jesus healed the sick?"

She frowned. "But of course, or I wouldn't be in church!"

They had drifted out to the vestibule after the services and were in a corner by themselves.

"Then you must believe what Jesus said about others being able to heal with faith in the Father."

"Of course," she said, remembering, " 'For where two or three are gathered in My name, there am I in the midst of them.' "

"Then would you mind if others prayed for your recovery?"

Hazel Wightt was flabbergasted. "Why should I mind being made well in Christ's name?"

The friend had called Dorothy Nelson and stated the problem. "Can your group help?"

"We can try," she said, deciding to have a go at it herself.

She put down the phone and concentrated. It took only a moment to get down to her levels and use the Screen of her Mind. She had the name, address, and the age. She apparently needed no more. She saw a woman with pale blue eyes and dark brown hair, quite incongruous for her years, and she knew with sudden conviction that she had locked into the right person.

"I put a light around her eyes and saw what I assumed to be cataracts drop away. I had the feeling, as remarkable as it was, that she was cured."

Three days later she got a second call from Hazel Wightt's friend. "It's a miracle!" he exclaimed. "Hazel can see again, and she is eternally grateful."

And so, trapped by her own feeling of obligation, Hazel Wightt had reluctantly agreed to bear witness to the wonders of Alpha, or whatever it was that had helped her.

She lived in a comfortable high-rise apartment for senior citizens. There was a sign on the lawn which said that neither children nor pets were allowed.

She seemed a little fidgety as she came to the door. She was a tall woman, with an ample bosom and a ruddy complexion. I was quick to note that she wore glasses, with gold rims.

She took them off as she showed us to a window seat overlooking the city, then offered us tea. It was all done in a grudging manner, and I found myself declining.

I had brought a tape recorder along, and she eyed it suspiciously. "I hope you're not going to use that," she said.

"Not if you don't want me to, but"—I paused—"with this, there is no danger of your being misquoted or misinterpreted."

"I don't like publicity," she said, and then threw an apologetic glance at Dorothy Nelson. "I agreed to do this out of gratitude for what you have done for me, but I really don't want to be in the spotlight."

I tried to mollify her. "If what I have been told is so, then your experience could very well be of help to other people."

She nodded curtly. "I'm aware of that, and I'm willing that you question me, so long as it is in good taste and not blown out of proportion. But please don't use the recording machine."

I failed to see the logic, but it was pointless to argue.

"Please tell me in your own words what happened regarding your eyesight."

She repeated pretty much what I had already heard, with added details about her visits to the doctor. "When I first went to the eye specialist, he told me I had cataracts, and not to worry, as my vision would improve after surgery. Meanwhile, he prescribed new glasses and told me to bring them in so he could check them over."

When the new glasses were finally ready, she tried them on, and had trouble seeing with them. She brought them back to the doctor, he tested them, then asked her to read from a chart with them on. She couldn't read very well. Tested with her old glasses, she read clearly. She looked up to catch a puzzled expression on the doctor's face. He examined her with a light held to her eyes, and when he had finished, she heard him muttering to himself, "I don't understand."

"May I ask what the trouble is, Doctor?" she asked.

"The trouble, my dear lady, is that you no longer have cataracts, and I have never had a similar case of spontaneous remission."

She looked up uncertainly, wondering whether to make a clean breast of it.

"Yes?" he said with a quick glance.

She came to a decision. "Doctor," she said, "do you believe in God?"

"Of course I believe in God," he said crustily.

"Do you believe God can heal?"

"I don't know why not if he's God." His voice was brusque and edged with impatience.

"Do you believe I could have been healed in God's name?"

The doctor gave her a curious look. She had been a patient of his for almost as many years as he had been a doctor. He knew her for a simple, straightforward person, an active churchgoer bound by convention, who would have sooner died than defy custom.

"The longer I live," the doctor said, "the more I realize there is another, greater force than man."

She was satisfied then that Dorothy Nelson, with God's help, had been the instrument of her amazing healing.

I heard her story through without comment, then said,

"Do you have any intention of meditating with Dorothy Nelson's prayer group?"

She gave me an impatient glance. "I have nothing to do with groups."

"I just thought that it might be an inspiration to them and others."

Her voice had an abrasive edge, and she looked at the wall clock.

"We have been hoping to get Mrs. Wightt to one of our meetings," Dorothy put in mildly.

Our hostess suddenly stood up and began to smooth the wrinkles out of her black silk dress. "I'll have to think that over," she said. "I'm not very good at appearances."

I had got to my feet and held out my hand. "I wish you luck," I said.

Her fingers barely touched mine. "I like very much to be by myself, not that I don't like people, but . . ." Her voice trailed off.

At the door, she had a few final words for me. "I trust you won't exaggerate. I know how reporters can be."

"How," I asked, "could anyone exaggerate what I have been told?"

Dorothy and I held our silence in the descending elevator. Finally, as we stepped out into the bright, sunny lobby, she sighed, "She is an old lady, set in her ways, and we shouldn't expect too much."

"At any rate," I said, "it makes an incredible story."

"Seeing her," Dorothy commented, "anybody would believe her. The story had to be dragged out of her."

The Hazel Wightt odyssey, unfortunately, did not end there. I inquired about her months later.

Dorothy Nelson was strangely pensive. "Oh, yes, I meant to drop you a note. The cataracts came back."

Immediately I was assailed with new doubts. "Had they ever gone?"

"Oh, yes." Her voice seemed tired. "But you can't block out love and withdraw from people when you have a chance to help without drawing something on yourself. Hazel Wightt forgot that God's law works both ways."

Dorothy was not discouraged by this experience. Her mother, living in Santa Monica, complained that her neck and shoulder were painfully out of position. Dorothy suggested she see a doctor. "Maybe later," she said, dismissing the idea.

While meditating a couple of days later, Dorothy recalled her mother's condition and took a look at her body on the Screen of the Mind. "I clearly saw the upper cervicals of her neck and spine out of alignment. In my levels, I adjusted her spine, bringing it into alignment."

Two hours later, she saw her mother. "You know, Dorothy," her mother said, "when I was getting dressed, I noticed that when I turned my head there was no pain." She smiled. "I couldn't help but wonder if you had worked on me."

"What time did the pain leave you?" Dorothy asked.

"Two hours ago," she said.

Asking Alpha teachers about Alpha was like asking Republicans about Eisenhower. Of course, they believed. Why else would they be teaching after taking the course?

"I wanted to change a few bad habits," said instructor Stewart Esposito, "and it changed my life."

Stew looked like a successful young insurance agent, and that's exactly what he was until Alpha struck.

I didn't know what I expected an Alpha teacher to look like, but it wasn't Stew. He was serious-faced, soberly dressed, and very determined. He made me think of that old ditty, "There's no one with endurance like the man who sells insurance."

He lived in Stamford, Connecticut, commuter distance from New York City, had an economics degree out of Cornell, was married, with a child, and still in his mid-twenties. He had everything going to fulfill the middle-class American dream of comfortable security. A few months out of college, he had sold a million dollars in life insurance, and was regarded by associates as a coming man. Hell, he was only twenty-five, and nobody could sell insurance like he could. He was making it. He was a blooming success. And he was also a nervous wreck.

He had migraine headaches, coffee jag, and he bit his nails.

"Everybody said I was a success, and I knew I was a mess." He exercised regularly, jogged daily, but it didn't help. "I'd get uncontrollably sleepy after lunch, pep myself up with coffee, and get tension headaches at four every afternoon."

He didn't look nervous or tense to me, rather stolid and placid, even phlegmatic.

But this was the new Stew Esposito. "The day I finished my mind class, I stopped drinking coffee." He looked up quizzically. "You say, 'big deal,' but I drank eight to ten cups a day to keep me alert for nighttime activity that I considered essential to the insurance business."

All these little miracles, and how were they done? Just by closing the eyes, going into the levels students talked about so glibly, and visualizing the horrible effects of the coffee? But hadn't he done this before? He must certainly have known what the coffee was doing to him or he wouldn't have been alert enough to have taken the course.

He had visualized himself, in class, as being fresh and wide awake, without coffee, and it had worked. He had imagined the bitter aftertaste of excessive coffee drinking, and it had worked. He had pictured himself as less nervous, more relaxed, and it had worked.

It had all happened in the Workshop, that wonderful dreamroom where all these dreams seemed to come true.

He had to keep up his autosuggestion—for what else was it?—just as he had to school himself every day, as an insurance man, to see so many prospects.

As he stopped drinking coffee, the daily headaches stopped. They were obviously an outgrowth of tension. Even when he did get an occasional headache, the course came in handy. "I would control the headache with a headache-removal technique demonstrated in the course. In your levels, you would recognize why you had your headache, tell yourself that you didn't want it, and put yourself in deep relaxation. There was no way you could hang onto it."

Not ever having seen the old Stew Esposito, I had nothing to compare the present one with. But he assured me he was a new person. "I haven't had any headaches for almost a year now, principally because my life has changed to a different level, with different values. I am a

calmer, more relaxed individual, at peace with myself."
Where once he had to make an effort at control, it now
came easier because he had formed new habit patterns.
"I don't drink coffee for stimulation because I don't need
it. I can stay up as long as I want and feel fresh the next
day. Sleep is never a problem."

It seemed to me that a grown man should have been
ashamed of biting his nails, and he had been. But he
couldn't stop, nevertheless. He nibbled at them nervously
till they were down to the quick. "This was a very real
torment for an adult man." He had sought all kinds of advice, but nobody could help him until he took the course
and was able to help himself. "You have no idea of the
significance of my being able to give up nail-biting."

And what had accomplished this wonder?

He applied a special reduction technique, reinforced by
positive visualization in his levels. It didn't happen all at
once. "The first day, I stopped biting my nails on my
first two fingers, still biting them on the other three, until, gradually reducing the number, I ran out of fingers to
bite."

As so often happened with mind graduates, the whole
family got into the act. Stew's young wife, Jackie, had
migraine headaches, too, and no wonder. Using Stew's
technique of getting into her own levels and disavowing
them, she soon got rid of her headaches. I couldn't help
thinking, though, even as Stew was discussing his own
metamorphosis, that just as some tension must have
rubbed off at home, his calm may now have done the
same.

Together the Espositos, in their levels, now started programming eighteen-month-old Stewart, Junior, and got
him on toilet-training, a matter he'd previously had little
interest in. They used the device of putting their infant son
on the Screen of their Minds, surrounding him with a
benevolent white light, and sending out the positive
thought that influenced his childish mind, regardless of
whether he was awake or asleep. "We dropped down to
our levels and really worked on him." They had a time
limit, and they made it. "It helped us enjoy our vaca-
tion," said the proud father.

Stew even kept his marriage serene with mind-training; fairly serene, that is. "We had marvelous experiences changing each other's moods through visual projection. If I got her angry, I'd put her on my Screen and calm her down, then keep her from holding a grudge." He smiled. "A very bad habit of hers."

Like so many students who went on to take the teacher course, he had been galvanized by his own experience. He wanted everybody to share his own awakening. It stimulated him to think that he could help others as he had been helped. Like Alexander Everett, he visualized a world where people would actually like one another. It could change the whole face of the globe as technology never could.

He recalled A. J. Jennings, a Fairfield, Connecticut, businessman, manager of an industrial plant, who had been as skeptical as anybody else until he saw Alpha-thinking work.

"He was able to alter the disposition of a younger, somewhat irrepressible member of his family by his own positive visualization, and project similar changes in personality to a business associate with a very sour outlook.

"In his mental Workshop," said Stew, "Jennings introduced an imaginary hypodermic needle, which he used to inject certain therapeutic medicines, mentally, of course, into the problem adolescent and business colleague."

I still couldn't even begin to grasp how thought transference of this nature could possibly work, yet Stew insisted that the man also got rid of his own hiccups by similarly injecting himself, mentally. It was obviously something that one would have to experience himself to credit. It was beyond anything the rational mind could begin to deal with. And its potential was endless.

In a more familiar area, if Esposito and Charlene Afremow were correct, why couldn't everybody program their children into positive pursuits, away from drugs, into doing their schoolwork and household chores promptly and becoming model children?

Esposito pointed out that Alpha graduates were doing it all the time. The Trog family in Waterbury, Connecticut, for instance. The parents were busy working, the father in real estate, the mother a social worker, and they had four children, three teen-age daughters and a son, ten-year-old Glen. Glen was having problems in school; his handwriting was hardly legible. He didn't seem able or willing to do anything about it (perhaps it was an attention-getter), and so Mother and Dad programmed him in their levels to improve his handwriting. Nothing was said on the conscious level. And, suddenly, in school one day, he started writing with a new legibility. There were other, more striking changes. Young Glen began to show remarkable psychic ability.

"Glen had become so psychic that once, while riding in the family car, he projected his mind into his home and described exactly what his mother, grandmother, and dog were doing at that very moment. It was all verified later."

Stew never seemed to run out of miracles. Some students cured themselves of insomnia, others lost excess weight, and others even learned to swim without being in water. There was an overweight girl who had lost weight without actually dieting. She had done it all in her head. Patricia Lamont, of New Canaan, Connecticut, had wanted to lose fifteen pounds, and she did it even though she had been on a 1,500-calorie-a-day diet for some time without losing a pound.

"Twice a day," said Stew, "Patricia went into her levels and programmed herself on the Screen of her mind. She looked at herself, as she was and as she wanted to be, and simply kept visualizing that anything she ate wouldn't turn to fat and that she would lose the weight she wanted —fifteen pounds."

Alexander Everett had told me I could become a genius, and I was beginning to consider the possibilities as Esposito regaled me with the story of a young Connecticut housewife named Sandra Muggett, who began to paint in the style of Van Gogh after sinking into the imaginary Workshop and visualizing the famous Dutch artist. "Van Gogh became very real and alive," said Stew. "He came over to her and took her hand and placed a drawing instrument in her hand and said, 'I want you to use your two fingers in this manner.' He put the two fingers together over the instrument. 'Go ahead and do your thing now,' he said.

"Well, the girl produced a work of art, unlike anything she had ever done before. It showed a distinct alteration from a flowing, perhaps feminine style, to the severe style of the great impressionist. According to people familiar with Van Gogh's landscapes and portraits, her work even resembled Van Gogh's."

How, I wondered, had she even in imagination presumed to tune into a painter dead these many years?

"We know," said Stew, "that it is relatively simple in Alpha to lock your mind into some living person you know. What Sandra did was quite unusual. But she did get the inspiration she wanted and it was all very real to her." In the subconscious state she had perhaps tuned into the same inspirational frequencies that Van Gogh may have been on.

Thought transference, which had puzzled me, presented no problems to one of the master architects of Alpha-Theta training, Dr. Robert Leichtman, a mind-oriented internist of the San Francisco suburb of Sausalito. "Kirlian photography suggests that when we change the thinking of man, we change his aura, the energy field emanating from living matter. Knowing from these pictures that the psychic extension of man actually exists, we are able to postulate that thoughts affecting the individual or his aura are not abstract or intangible things. They have obvious form and are evidently made of subtle matter, capable of moving from a projective mind level to the subconscious level of another."

Differing from Alexander, the physician considered it obvious that thought transference could be either positive or negative. Phenomena had no morals. "We can't change the laws of nature, we can only adapt to them, just as we do to electricity or the law of gravity. If the potential receiver remains calm, in control of his own emotions and in mastery of himself, there is little possibility of his becoming a victim of mental malpractice, since few chinks exist in a well-integrated personality. However, emotionally upset, fraught with fear and anxiety, he is vulnerable to the negative thoughts of others."

The physician laughed as he explained how thought transference could work beneficially, and in doing so provided an explanation for A. J. Jennings and his hypodermic needle.

He had directed his Alpha-Theta mind to an office

secretary who had complained of disfiguring facial hives whenever she became acutely nervous. The hives caused her such embarrassment that she was planning to cancel a trip to Reno.

"With all this mind power of yours," she said, "why can't you do something for me?"

"I'll try," said Dr. Leichtman as she left the room.

At noon that day, he visualized her, saw her face clearly with the hives, and began mentally applying a cortisone ointment which medical experience told him was beneficial for this disorder. He did this for two or three minutes, with the conviction that the treatment was in the process of completely removing the hives. There was no doubt in his mind.

A half hour later, the excited secretary came rushing into his office. "They're going, they're going," she cried, pointing to the diminishing signs of the rash on her face.

The doctor nodded matter-of-factly. "But of course."

She gave him a quizzical look. "Were you working on me at noon?"

"Why do you ask?"

"Because I felt somebody's fingers stroking my face at that time."

Listening to this story, I wondered what influence, if any, the cortisone had played in the suggestive process.

"Do you think," I asked, "that having cortisone in your subconscious mind somehow materialized it onto her face?"

"Hardly," he said. "But what it most likely did was to focus my power of mind in a way that it traditionally knew to be most constructive."

"In other words," I said, "you added the necessary ingredient of expectancy."

We had discussed the conscious and the subconscious, but Dr. Leichtman introduced a new factor, the superconscious mind, which he described as a more powerful dimension of the mind than the subconscious. It seemed like semantics since I was sure that the various functions of the mind overlapped just as Beta, Alpha and Theta frequently manifested themselves together in some imaginative burst of inspiration.

"Not true," said Dr. Leichtman. "In the superconscious

27

state, which can be reached through the relaxed detachment of meditation on the higher self, the individual becomes aware of his true identity and in this new realization contacts his immortal soul."

I looked at him doubtfully. "How do you prove one intangibility by another?"

"By function and by result," he said, "both tangible factors in scientific experience."

I recalled the pathologist who had looked down on the dissecting table and mordantly asked a student, "Show me the soul in this cadaver."

Leichtman laughed. "The soul had left, for the soul is the life force animating the body. The soul expresses the love behind emotions and the wisdom behind the mind, transcending the subconscious mind."

The line of demarcation still didn't appear clear to me.

"In this transcendent state," the doctor went on, "there is an expansion of consciousness in which the individual merges his life force with the oneness of the universe and recognizes, perhaps for the first time, that he can count on this universe for support anytime he needs it."

It seemed like a pretty tall order. "Is he in Alpha or Theta at this time?" I asked.

"The brainwaves automatically conform. They are an index of thought, not thought itself. And usually in the Alpha state there is also some Theta mixed in."

I still did not see how it was any different from the subconscious mind.

He searched about in his mind for a distinctive example and came up with a youthful veteran of the Vietnamese war.

"He had been off drugs for a year and a half before he came to me, but despite a long bout of psychotherapy, he was living with fear of his own fragility and what he might do to himself at any time."

He had become interested in Leichtman's class on self-improvement because he had fallen in love and was planning to marry. Knowing his own insecurity, he was hoping to acquire the strength needed for this new responsibility.

"Why didn't he put himself up on the Screen of his Mind," I asked, "and visualize himself as the perfect bridegroom?"

"It isn't quite that simple, particularly in his case," said the doctor, "since he had been trying to improve his self-image for months and he had nobody else to turn to."

With drugs and without, he had felt desperately alone, at the mercy of forces beyond his control. The soul had little relevance to him. Now Leichtman was explaining that the soul was an infinite power upon which he could benevolently draw. But it still meant nothing, until the doctor described his own experience.

"In deepest meditation, I sense myself surrounded by an infinite lighted presence, an ocean of white light shining on me, with a radiating, loving, nurturing quality. As I open myself to this light, approaching it with an attitude of trust and reverence, I feel this light loving me and the essence of my being merges with its radiance."

And how had the young veteran done?

"Drawing on the lighted presence in his own meditation, he identified the light he saw with himself and suddenly realized this light was a true reflection of his soul."

After the meditation he approached Leichtman and there was a smile on his face. He had transcended the subconscious, entering a superconscious level which revealed the oneness of man and his universe.

"For the first time in my life," he said, "I am not afraid. I realize that I have a companion who is a part of me, just as I am part of him, and I shall never again feel alone. I have somebody to turn to, somebody who cares, somebody who knows about me just as I know about him, and somebody who loves me as I love him."

I looked at Leichtman, still a little doubtful. "And it all came out of this white light?"

"No, it was his transcending feeling about the light in his superconscious state. He was moved to tears by his heartfelt conviction that there is a common source, a mainspring and reason for his being."

It seemed to me that something was still missing.

The physician smiled. "Naturally," he said, "for by its very nature, a superconscious experience defies verbal definition. It comes as a revelation, it moves the individual to a full awareness of his place in the universe, his true purpose of life, and a discovery of his own uniqueness. Some, like Paul on the road to Damascus, experience this spontaneously and it brings a permanent transformation."

Had the young veteran been hypnotized into this exalted state?

"Not at all," said Leichtman. "He went beyond himself in communing with his own soul. In hypnosis the individual never gets beyond the outer perimeter of his own personality. He can only dredge up that which is in his conscious and subconscious level."

Some self-styled scientists argued that the key to the Alpha brainwave—or for that matter, Delta, Theta, and Beta—were the Biofeedback devices which involved the use of electroencephalograph machines, enabling the subject to know how many brainwaves he was producing per second. In Beta, said these mechanists, the EEG recorded fourteen to twenty-eight cycles, or circuits, per second, though it often spiked upward to fifty or more under stress. Beta, they said, manifested itself in ordinary sensory situations, in anxiety, fear, frustration and anger, and was associated with measured consideration of everyday problems. It was a highly unglamorous state.

In Alpha, as the mind level deepened, the brainwaves dropped to eight to thirteen cycles. In Theta, the drowsy state, the brainwave patterns slowed from four to seven cycles per second, and in Delta, from aproximately .5 to three.

I still had no clear idea how the reputed wonders of Alpha could be effectively harnessed. Certainly, society could hardly survive a swarm of laymen wandering about diagnosing illnesses they had no right to treat even if correct in their assumptions.

I looked about for something more substantial to go on. What were the scientists doing? Eagerly I turned up at UCLA, the University of California at Los Angeles, for a series of informed lectures on "Alpha—the Wave of the Future?" I listened to Dr. Barbara Brown, chief of experimental physiology, Veterans Administration Hospital, Los Angeles, and Dr. Joseph Kamiya, research specialist, Langley Porter Neuropsychiatric Institute, San Francisco. Dr. Brown reported that the brain had approximately ten to twenty billion brain cells, all interconnected, and that these cells produced electric signals, detected by the electroencephalograph, of fluctuating frequency when firing together. Her data indicated an altered state of consciousness associated with Alpha production that did not necessarily induce a dramatic behavioral change. She saw no scientific correlation between extrasensory perception ability and brainwaves when, on an observer's level, I saw hardly anything else.

She had reservations about who engaged in Alpha-wave feedback, specifically excluding depressive neurotics, epileptics, mental cases, heavy marijuana users, and heroin addicts, claiming their conditions might actually worsen.

Training in Alpha feedback, Kamiya reported, increased the susceptibility to hypnosis, with some having a perfect recall of an object after it had been removed. The relationship between experimenter and subject—and I presumed teacher and student—affected Alpha production. If the relationship was warm, Alpha activity increased; if cold or hostile, it decreased. Meanwhile, in the exciting laboratory of life, a whole new vista of awareness was opening up, extending even to the dream world.

With Alpha-Theta meditation, many, like Bill Schwartz of Milwaukee's Meditation Institute, sought to explore this subconscious wasteland with new awareness. "At night, the subconscious mind is always talking to us," Schwartz tells his students. "To understand dreams, we have to understand the language of the subconscious, and this may be like learning a foreign language because the subconscious talks to us in symbols and other forms of nonverbal communication. The subconscious often uses places that are familiar to us, people who are familiar to us, things that we know of or have heard of. But to find the meaning, we frequently have to go beyond the cast and the surface action and get into the plot, the mood and direction of the action, as you would with a movie you were watching. Relate that plot to something that is occurring in your life, which you can use to give yourself direction or to help understand yourself, others and events you are currently involved with."

Bill Schwartz believed, like many, that creative people were normally in Alpha and Theta and, drowsy or asleep, were at least as inventive as in the waking state. He cited a dream by Elias Howe. "Elias was on the verge of putting the sewing machine together, but the last knotty problem was how to thread the needle. He tried the conventional way from the top, but it didn't work. One night, he went to bed late, with the problem very much on his mind. He had a dream that night, in which he was in a jungle (the labyrinth of his confused mind) and the natives captured him at spearpoint and took him to their leader.

"The leader said, 'Elias Howe, you have until morning to invent the sewing machine. If you don't, we will toss you into a big pot, boil you, and then eat you.' Morning came, and still no sewing machine.

"The irate chief," Schwartz continued with the dream, "ordered his men to fire their spears at the hapless inventor. As they held their arms poised, ready to thrust their spears into him, he noticed the lower tips of the spears had a hole in them. He woke up immediately, knowing how to thread the sewing machine, from the bottom rather than from the top of the needle—just like the spearheads."

Robert Louis Stevenson also used his dreams to produce his most memorable tales. "In one of his dreams, a man, running from the police, ducked into an alley and reached into his back pocket. He pulled out a flask, drank from it, and instantly became a completely altered person, in nature and appearance. This was the beginning of Dr. Jekyll and Mr. Hyde."

Schwartz encouraged his students to dream-sleep on their everyday problems even as they meditated. One student, a natural gas dealer, was confronted with the problem of storing thirty thousand gallons of gas for a cold weather emergency, not wanting to buy a giant tank when he needed it for only the two coldest weeks of the year.

"So, in meditation, he used the technique of requesting a dream for the purpose of solving his problem. On this relaxing level, he slipped into a light slumber and the programmed dream obligingly came through. He saw some very small gas tanks flying past him like rocket ships, and there were thirty of them. It added up to thirty thousand gallons. As he wondered what this meant, the answer came to him. He was to buy thirty one-thousand-gallon tanks and sell one to thirty different customers, so they could store their gas on their own premises. He proceeded to buy the tanks immediately, not only solving the storage problem but saving a considerable price rise, as the cost of the tanks went up the next day."

Just as dreams were a language of the subconscious, meditation with its symbolism was a form of intellectual shorthand, controlling emotions outside the province of the rational mind. "Expecting the intellect to handle emotional problems is like your right hand guiding your feet," said the youthful Schwartz. "For the subconscious mind is the seat of our emotional nature."

With practice, the student would acquire sufficient detachment in his Workshop to examine his inner self in his deeper levels of the mind. Meanwhile, Schwartz counseled students: "Picture someone else in your shoes, acting and reacting as you normally do. This could be a stranger or somebody you know. Imagine until it is reality and you see this person—you—clearly and with detachment."

At this level, the individual can discriminate between what he is and what he is expected to be. "He is no longer torn by an uneasy image created by others; personality conflicts blocking tranquillity and growth are ended."

Bill Schwartz had emerged from his own self-appraisal bloody but unbowed. He had been a floundering businessman when he first saw himself on the Screen of the Mind, and it had made him an almost instant success, as he visualized a new purposeful self-image. But in creating this image, he soon turned his back on his newfound success to become, first, an instructor with Alexander Everett, then a teacher on his own. "As it is within," said he, "so shall it be without."

I didn't see why the beginner couldn't take a direct look at himself just as easily.

"It's a matter of learning detachment," Schwartz said. "We generally think our situation is worse than anyone else's, that no one is ever as bad as we are, so we hesitate to talk about it frankly. But relating the experience to someone else, we feel free to question this individual. And he as freely discusses his secret fears and drives, which of course are our own.

"On this deeper level, we readily replace negativity with a positive image. We do not have to change our values— just the way we act out our values. One believes in God, piously going to church. Another believes as deeply, without church, but in loving his fellow man."

The word symbol *psychosomatic* was an illustration of how things got turned around negatively. "We have the *psyche* and the *soma*, the mind and the body working together, a very positive concept. But we intellectually attach to it a connotation of sickness, whereas it could just as easily be psychosomatic health. The subconscious doesn't think in words, and so we use pictures to eliminate negative symbols and promote the positive. Einstein pointed out, 'Imagination is more important than knowledge.' "

The individual has an intellect and a body, desires and fears, but, more, he is a center of awareness, establishing clearly his identity and purpose. "This center is in touch with all that he is and does."

On the conscious level, there were obvious obstacles. "Words have different meanings to different people, and some emotions, resentment and hostility, block off communication. But at the deep mind level of Alpha-Theta there are no barriers, and this may be why it works."

The higher intelligence reaches out from this center of awareness to the higher intelligence of others. "In this dimension, any physical problem will show up gray to black, depending on its severity. At this level, on their imaginary screens, I tell students, mentally, to make a correction, applying remedies from their Workshops, or doing whatever else they feel should be done. And they can do it to themselves just as easily as to another."

Chapter 3

When the Pupil Is Ready

If it worked, I wanted to know more about it and let other people know about it, if they so desired. And so I decided to take the course, even though, as I understood, many of the scientifically minded researchers had never had the curiosity, or confidence, to test their own Alpha output, with or without Biofeedback machines.

I had invited a few friends to take the course with me, to check their reactions with my own. Actresses Anne Francis and Eve Bruce, former model Linda Lockwood, and Hollywood casting director Ralph Winters had been as eager as I for the experience.

"What can it do for me?" Ralph had asked.

"They say it improves memory, helps you concentrate, and makes you more creative."

"So what are we waiting for?"

"You have to be expectant," Alexander Everett had said, and Anne Francis was certainly that. The glamorous blonde star was as excited as if she were going to her first high school prom.

"Isn't it wonderful to have this opportunity?" she said as we drove together to class.

I gave her a sidelong glance. She seemed to have everything—beauty, health, a lovely home and children, an ongoing career. "What can it possibly do for you?"

She frowned a moment. "It's more what I can do for others. Edgar Cayce said you get to heaven on the arms of the people you've helped."

"And how do you propose to do this?"

She laughed engagingly. "I hope for some new awareness that will give me direction."

"Why is it," I asked, "that people who seem to have everything are so often dissatisfied?"

She had thought about it. "Once a person attains the usual goals, he discovers so often that success hasn't filled the void. Look at all the successful people on drugs and booze, too frightened by the prospect of living to face life."

I looked at her curiously as we drew up to the class site, Los Angeles' Ambassador Hotel. "Perhaps we're doing the same in taking this course."

"We're jumping into something, not out of it."

Students were already milling about inside. Alexander stood outside the lecture room, chatting. He greeted us with an easy smile. I couldn't help thinking that he looked more like a banker than a mind-merchant. He was conservatively clad in suit and tie, harmonizing with his British correctness. He was fifty or so, but looked younger. There were no lines in the ruddy face.

"Welcome," he drawled, thrusting out a hand.

As Anne Francis went off to register, I gave him a little preview of my intentions. "Any book on the Alpha wave," I said, "should feature a do-it-yourself program, since the course may be too expensive for some."

He waved a hand in the direction of a group of young people lined up with Anne. "At least, when somebody pays for the course, you know they want to do something about themselves. Some of these kids had to make sacrifices to be here."

"In many communities," I pointed out, "qualified teachers won't be available."

He shook his head. "Even if they read a book and understood the fundamentals, they will still miss the flow of energy from other students."

I looked at him questioningly. "You are saying that people in Alpha actually produce a physical energy?"

"There is no miracle about psychic healings, visualizing the future, or creating. We are all fields of electromagnetic energy, and in this flow of energy, the more sensitive we are, the better the transmitter and receiver we are."

I peered into the room and saw some fifty potential transmitters. I took the only chair available, sitting directly in front of a lovely girl with long hair and sparkling blue eyes. She gave me a perfunctory nod. To my left, I noticed a middle-aged couple loaded down with blankets and pillows. As Alexander took his place by a large blackboard, facing the class, my eyes roamed about the long, narrow room. The students were of all ages and types. The younger men were in sweaters and sport shirts, the older ones wore suits and ties. The younger women, like the girl behind me, seemed disposed to slacks; the older were in dresses and skirts. I spotted a few familiar faces: actors' agent Ernie Dade, Eve Bruce, Linda Lockwood, and Ralph Winters, of course and one or two others.

Alexander's voice carried clearly. "All of us, except for a handful of natural-born geniuses, don't really know how we think, except, vaguely, that it has to do with that gray matter we call the brain. We don't realize that every cell of the body has an intelligence of its own, and that by becoming aware of this intelligence we can send messages to these cells and to the cells of other intelligences."

I looked around the room and saw that the only people who seemed to grasp what he was saying were the few graduates he had brought along to help moderate test cases on the final class day.

"Today"—he paused—"you will be introduced to a technique which will enable you to use the ninety percent of your mind you haven't been using. Great inner changes will take place in all of you here. They will come about slowly, imperceptibly, so that on the fourth and last day, when you all go into your test cases, you will be amazed by your own awareness, by your ability to look into the minds and bodies of people you have never seen. And above all, to look clearly into yourself, so that you will be making contact with your true self for the first time." His eyes seemed to reach everybody in the room. "I want you to regard these next four days not as a class but as an experience, as an open sesame to the wonders of boundless living."

A swift ripple of interest ran through the class.

In a cordial tone, he invited everybody to make themselves comfortable. "Sit anywhere you like, on the floor if you prefer." His eyes took in the middle-aged man with the blankets and pillows. "You look," he said pleasantly, "as if you have come well-prepared."

The man looked back almost defensively. He was short and stocky, with heavy jowls and a sallow face. He looked tired. "I was told that even if I slept through the sessions it wouldn't make any difference."

As the class laughed, Alexander smiled easily. "As a matter of fact," he said, "you may do better. I will be appealing to your subconscious mind, and that's where the big changes will be taking place." He waved a hand at the floor. "Be my guest."

The man sat down against the wall, comfortably propped himself against a pillow, and motioned his wife to join him. They put a blanket down, practically under Alexander's feet. His nose wrinkled for an instant. He looked as if he were about to say something, but instead moved leisurely toward the center of the room.

"Since we will be closely associated for a few days, it might be a good idea if each person stood and gave his name. Let's start with the first row."

Yawning, the little man rose and said, "Lennie Weitz, at your service."

He sat down, and his wife got up, darting an aggrieved look at the imperturbable Alexander.

Anne Francis rose in her blonde loveliness, our only celebrity.

Then with the roster completed, a quizzical smile crossed Alexander's face. "How many can remember the names they just heard?"

"All the names?" a voice asked incredulously.

"All the names, in the order given."

Not a single hand went up.

"Before the course is completed, all of you should be able to do this easily."

There was a murmur of subdued laughter, and a few students looked around uncertainly.

"Now I want all of you to relax," Alexander began. "Make sure that your arms and legs are not crossed so that you may better relax." He took a deep breath. "All right, everybody close your eyes, and keep them closed for this eight-minute training cycle. However, if you feel you must open your eyes, you may if you wish. Also, if

38

you want to move, scratch, or even clear your throat, you may do so."

I closed my eyes, thinking that a loose rein probably helped keep things relaxed.

"With your eyes closed, take some deep breaths. Breathe slowly and deeply, and every time you breathe out, feel yourself becoming more and more relaxed. Just let your body go and relax. Breathe in and out and relax."

The word *relax* was spoken slowly, with emphasis.

I slid an eye open and glanced around the room. Everybody was breathing in and out slowly, with their lids shut. The girl behind me looked as if she were in a trance.

"To help you reach a deeper and more inward level of mind, I shall count from twenty-one down to one. On every descending number you will feel yourself going deeper and more inward, nearer to the very source of your being."

This sounded very much like the countdown induction of the hypnotist, but I remembered Alexander saying that only the techniques to relax the body were similar and that hypnosis was basically authoritarian while mind-training was subjective.

The countdown proceeded slowly:

"Twenty-one—twenty—nineteen: Feel yourself going deeper.

"Eighteen—seventeen—sixteen: Go deeper within.

"Fifteen—fourteen—thirteen: Deeper and deeper.

"Twelve—eleven—ten: Feel yourself going inward.

"Nine—eight—seven: Go more inward.

"Six—five—four: Inner and inner.

"Three—two—one."

He stopped for a moment. "You are now at a much deeper and more inward level of mind, near to the very source of your being. To further tune into your inner levels of mind, visually pick out a passive scene from nature, any scene that you find serenely beautiful and relaxing. Just become calm, still, at peace, and see yourself mentally within your passive scene. Reach out and feel the vibrant life forces of nature that surround you and feel in perfect tune with your inner levels of mind."

I had counted down to myself, like the others, I

imagined, and I visualized the rolling waves breaking on the surf outside my Malibu window. I felt very much at peace, except for a slow, rhythmic buzzing on my left. I opened my eyes toward the direction of the sound. Lennie Weitz, comfortably camped on the floor, with a blanket up to his chin, was peacefully snoring.

"Poor Lennie," I thought, "sleeping away all that money."

I saw Alexander frown for a moment, then move on.

"You are now in tune with your inner levels—*relax*. . . . Every time you hear me mention the word *relax*, your body, brain, and mind [an interesting distinction, I thought] will become completely passive and relaxed. As you continue to relax your body, brain, and mind, you will become more aware and alert at your inner conscious levels.

"You will continue to follow instruction at all levels of mind, including the outer conscious level. You will repeat to yourself certain positive phrases for your own benefit and progress."

Significantly, perhaps, the *you* now became the first person singular, *I*, and control apparently passed to the student. "Repeat after me, 'I am continually thinking positive thoughts that make me successful, happy, and prosperous.

" 'I am using more and more of my mind and using it in such a special manner that I have full and complete domination over all my senses and faculties at every level of the mind, including the outer conscious level.

" 'I am also using my positive thinking to bring me the understanding and awareness that I desire, so that my increasing mental faculties may be used to serve humanity better. In fact, every day in every way, I am getting better and better.' "

Alexander now prepared the class to leave its levels.

"Remember, anytime you enter your levels, you receive benefits both physically and mentally. You may also use your levels not only to help yourself but also your friends and relatives, and any other human being who needs help.

"Always use your deeper and inner levels of the mind in a constructive and creative manner for all that is good, honest, and positive. Never use these levels of the mind to do harm to yourself or any other person. If this is your intention, you will find you will not be able to function within your levels."

I was not sure at this point what these levels were, since my inquiring mind was restlessly trying to determine what was going on.

"In a moment, I will ask you to open your eyes. You will be wide awake in perfect health, feeling revitalized and refreshed, and in tune with life."

I glanced around the room. Lennie Weitz was sitting up, rubbing his eyes. Actress Eve Bruce appeared enthralled, Ralph Winters intrigued, and Anne Francis seemed almost hypnotized. The precocious teen-ager behind me was in an expansive mood, her smile warmer and more direct. But to my critical eye, aside from Lennie, nobody seemed conspicuously revitalized, and the reason for his fresh, shiny face was obvious. He'd had a good sleep.

It was time for our first coffee break. Ralph Winters introduced me to a hawk-faced man of thirty or so, with a pretty girl. He was wildly waving his arms.

"It's an outrage, that's what, paying a hundred and fifty dollars for something like that. It's hypnosis, that's all it is."

"Don't forget," his girl friend chimed in, "you paid for me, too."

"Don't remind me," he said. He turned to me abruptly. "What do you make of it?"

Ralph Winters had made a deprecating noise. "Joe's a writer," he said, "and a little impulsive."

"It's a little early for judgments, Joe," I said, "but maybe, like the man said, it'll calm you down."

"I don't need calming down," snapped Joe.

"Give it time," said Winters soothingly. "We've only just begun."

"I like it better," said Joe, unreconciled, "when the Carpenters are singing it."

"And how about that character sleeping through it all?" his girl friend said.

"He's better off than he knows," Joe growled.

Ralph glanced at his watch and called for the check. "Time to go now."

"Are you going back?" I asked Joe.

He heaved his heavy shoulders. "I have to, I paid for it."

Alexander was ready and waiting. "Any questions?"

A lone hand went up—Joe's. "What does all this stuff have to do with Alpha?"

Alexander good-naturedly brushed aside the grumpiness. "Once you have learned through our technique to get down into your levels, you will be in Alpha, and perhaps some Theta, if you're a good little boy."

Joe bristled. "How will we know, without a Biofeedback machine?"

"You'll know by the way you suddenly function, knowing what people are going to say before they say it, tuning in on friends at a distance, wanting to help people. The Biofeedback is only a yardstick, and you can't carry it with you, like you do your own head."

He hesitated, then seemed to come to a decision. "I think it's time for a little demonstration of what mind-training can do." He held up a blunt end of white chalk. "Beginning with the first row, I want each person to give me a word. I will write it on the blackboard, and then, with my back to the board—blindfolded, if you like—I will repeat each word in the order given."

He pointed to the first row.

"Railroad," a student promptly said.

I was seventh, and gave the word *book*.

And so it went until he had chalked fifty words on the blackboard, in vertical columns. Even though I had schooled my own memory so that I seldom took notes, I had the feeling Alexander had given himself a large order. But he seemed confident.

"Railroad," he began, which surprised no one, and ran off six words quickly, all correctly. Then, looking at me, he gave the seventh, "book." He faltered only once on number twenty-five, starting to give the twenty-sixth, then corrected himself. He ran off the next twenty-five words rapidly. He had done it perfectly.

He took his success in stride. "After lunch," he said with

a sly glance for Joe, "I'll show you how you can do as much. It's all mind-training, a very simple technique."

His tone turned briskly professorial. "Now, close your eyes and direct your attention to your eyelids, in particular the little muscles around your eyes. Just relax these tiny muscles and let them go, and feel this relaxation moving like a wave, slowly downward throughout your body."

I had been listening too intently, perhaps, for instead of feeling relaxed, I found myself fidgeting under the restraint of keeping my eyes closed and relaxing an eyelid I had suddenly become aware of.

I opened my eyes and caught Alexander's gaze.

"Don't try to relax," he said. "Allow your mind to drift, casually and detached, unconcerned with the results of concentration, as you tell yourself to relax. It will happen without any noticeable effort."

Alexander let his eyes wander lazily around the classroom. "Now direct your sense of awareness to the top of your head, the scalp, to the actual skin that covers the head. You will notice a feeling of warmth, the blood circulating, the fine pulsation, then relax the scalp completely, let it go."

From the scalp, Alexander moved to the face, cheeks, jaw, and throat—the vocal chords themselves, the ligaments and tendons, with the suggestion that the student cause the tissues and cells to function in a healthy manner.

Not being a pathologist, I could only imagine what these tissues looked like, and they came up pink and clear.

The downward progression continued through the shoulders, chest, lungs, heart, knees, toes, and the soles of the feet, all coupled with total relaxation and rhythmic deep breathing.

Alexander now introduced the colors of the rainbow, symbolizing the different stages of relaxing into our levels. As he relaxed physically, the student saw the color Red. At the color Orange, he concentrated on his emotions and mastering these emotions. With Yellow, he calmed his mind, drinking in beautiful scenes from nature. "Whenever you visualize the color Yellow, calm and still your mind."

With Green, the student visualized inner peace, and Blue was the color for love. With Purple, he saw himself on the Screen, and with Violet, he entered another phase of his levels. After the color descent came the countdown from twenty-one, with the suggestion that with every descending number he sink deeper into his levels and nearer the source of his being.

With the others, I then entered my passive scene from nature. I visualized the surf pounding the beach as I sat relaxed on a rock in the sand, smelling the salt spray and feeling the tang of the breeze against my cheek.

Initially, my mind was as restless as the wind. But as I forced myself to visualize Red, I saw a red apple and saw myself biting it. With Yellow, I basked in the golden sunshine and felt a luxurious warmth creep over me. I came to the Green of the forest and felt myself sinking more and more into a state of euphoria. With Blue, I saw the clear azure sky, Purple, the twilight, and with Violet, a misty haze that gradually merged into the endless sea.

By the time we approached the countdown, my mental processes had slowed and I was feeling rather than thinking. I supposed I was in my levels. The countdown was almost superfluous at this stage. I kept visualizing steps as we came down from twenty-one, and felt my attention wandering. The sameness of visualizing one step after another made the whole exercise a chore, so that I became conscious of the procedure, defeating the projected goal of removing conscious thinking. With the passive scene from nature, I again shed conscious thought and began to feel the well-being I associated with nature. Obviously, the overall procedure was a little elaborate for my needs, and thereafter I eliminated the countdown and went right from Alexander's rainbow to my nature scene.

Opening my eyes, mentally rubbing out the spray of the sea, I was back in the reality of the classroom. I sat there for a while, trying to analyze what it meant, at this stage, to be in my levels. I had felt my mind drifting lazily, free of tension and purpose, free of my body.

At luncheon with Ralph Winters and Anne Francis, I observed, "I feel as if I'd had a restful sleep."

Their experience was similar to mine, except that they

44

had visualized without a conscious break, but then they didn't have a split role of observer and participant.

Alexander had assured us that we should take each step in stride, and I supposed the opportunity to be a genius would present itself soon enough.

I had been impressed by Alexander's memory demonstration but considered this a personal quirk of his. Nevertheless, it seemed a wonderful quality for an actor.

"How'd you like to remember your lines like old Alexander?" I asked.

Anne shrugged. "Most actors have their own techniques."

"Can you imagine what collegians could do with this boning up for exams?"

We passed the table where Joe was grumpily paying his bill. He gave us a jaundiced look. "What a crock," he said.

"Think Blue," said Ralph.

Alexander was ready for his lesson in memory control. He took us into our levels, with the rainbow sequence and the twenty-one countdown, and suggested we mentally create a large screen some distance away. "Make this screen as large as you like, any color you like. Design it exactly as you want it to be, for this is the Screen of the Mind."

Mine was a large screen, in Cinerama's living color.

On this Screen of the Mind we were to visualize ten pictures in sequence. "This practice will increase your ability to visualize and imagine, and so help your memory. Associate each picture with a corresponding number and word.

"One, Tea; picture a glass of iced tea with a large number 1 painted on its side.

"Two, Noah; visualize an old man with a beard, and animals entering the Ark 2 by 2.

"Three, May; the month of May, a country scene with a clump of 3 tall trees.

"Four, Ray; 4 rays of light shining through a window.

"Five, Law; a policeman with Badge #5 on his chest.

"Six, Jaw; a wrestler with a large rugged jaw, with 6 teeth jutting out.

"Seven, Key; a heavily engraved gold key in the shape of a 7.

"Eight, Fee; large price tag for 8 million dollars.

"Nine, Bay; water surrounded by land in the shape of a 9.

"Ten; your own 10 toes."

I ran over the list, surprised that I could remember each in order visually, but still wondering how this had helped Alexander recall fifty words at random. But he had moved on to the Screen of the Mind as a project solver.

"Just look at the imperfections in the black frame, running through your daily life at home, the office, and in public. Analyze yourself in detail, observe how you act and react to other people. See what you are doing wrong. Visualize everyday situations. For example, see yourself driving, notice your reaction when another car cuts in front of you. How often do you put the other driver in the wrong? Now the gas station. See yourself filling up your car with gas and notice how the attendant pokes along, not even bothering to clean the windshield. How do you react? How do you react at the supermarket when there is a long line at the cash register? Next, see yourself at work. Are you giving your best, or just enough to get along? How do you react to management decisions for the betterment of the company that compels you to work harder?

"Select a friend and bring him to the Screen of the Mind. Do you force your views on this person, without giving him a chance to express yourself? See yourself at home with your family. Are you reasonable, critical, demanding? Do you think your wife or son's point of view unimportant and that no one in the family knows as much as you? Consider these situations on the Screen of the Mind. Be honest with yourself."

There flashed a distant scene of an editor telling an aspiring feature writer that he lacked the newspaper's knack of doing things, and of the dejected slope of his shoulders as he turned away. With a little encouragement, perhaps the young writer might have made it. And now, unpredictably, after all these years, it was on that editor's Screen of the Mind. Next, some teen-agers, laughing riotously as they careened their car past a startled motorist. He cussed them out roundly, and nervously slammed on his brakes, feeling his stomach tighten up and a dull headache forming. Why hadn't I waved back and sent pleasant thoughts?

Alexander's voice cut in. "Now you will make a change. I shall count from one to three. At three, you will change the frame from black to white and allow a shower of white light to pour over your whole body. As this white light immerses you, feel an actual change taking place and watch yourself become a different person on the Screen of the Mind. Let this white light completely cleanse and purify you. Release your negativity, forgive, and give forth only that which is good. You will now act and react toward your fellow man in a considerate and loving manner. Feel this white light moving through you and making you a better and more beautiful being. Always see yourself on the Screen of the Mind surrounded by a white light and a white frame, in a state of wholeness and perfection."

I had no problem visualizing a white light, though my own features seemed indistinct, and I had the eerie feeling I was actually seeing somebody else. "To help you reinforce this new self-image, create a portrait of yourself as you wish to be on the Screen of the Mind. Etch in a general outline of how you feel you should look. Start by painting your face. Paint your skin with a bright, healthy glow, your cheeks reflecting good circulation. Define your nose and nostrils, and the cheekbones; keep the jaw line firm. Make your forehead broad and powerful; bring in a smile as you paint your mouth. Make your teeth white, clean, and straight, reflecting the care you give them. Make the eyes sparkling, bright, alert, shining with understanding, friendliness, confidence. Mentally paint in eyebrows that indicate your ability to concentrate, expressive so they can be raised in question. Define your ears as instruments for accurate hearing. Moving to the top of your head, paint in your hair. Choose it long or short, conservative or freer in style, looking alive and well-groomed. Choose whatever dress style pleases you, and the colors that suit you best. Step back and observe your new portrait. You can always modify it, since you are, as in life, your own creator. Touch up, add, or change anything you wish whenever you look at yourself on the Screen of the Mind."

And now, slowly, Alexander proceeded to take us out of our levels.

My eyes fell on Lennie Weitz. He was yawning as his wife bundled together the blankets and pillows.

Alexander watched a moment, then caught himself. "Any questions?"

I raised my hand. "I still don't see how you called off those fifty words in a row?"

"Visually I have memorized one hundred consecutive word associations."

"But how did you get *railroad* out of a glass of tea?"

"I visualized a glass of tea with a large 1 painted on it, served in a *railroad* dining car."

"And my word, *book?*"

He turned to the board. "As you called off your word, associating 7 with Key, I flashed a picture of a key opening a book on the Screen of my Mind."

Just memorizing the word associations seemed an insuperable task to me.

"And you never mix them up?"

"Not in my levels." He smiled. "Can you recall the ten words I gave you?"

I closed my eyes and visualized them quickly down to my ten toes. As a former editor had once said, "One picture is worth a thousand words."

Chapter 4

We March On

As I hesitated before the Ambassador, noticing a traffic officer, Anne said, "Oh, he won't mind if you turn into the driveway from the center lane. There's no traffic."

Newly susceptible to suggestion, I made my turn, and in my rearview mirror saw an all too familiar flashing red signal. "Oh, no, he won't mind!"

The officer got out of his machine slowly and peered into the open window. As his eyes moved to Anne, I saw a glint of recognition.

He scanned my license, then handed it back with a smile. "Seeing as you don't live in the city, I'll let you go this time. But don't let it happen again."

It was the first time I had ever been stopped for a moving violation and escaped without a ticket. "He recognized you from your movies," I decided as he drove off.

"That had nothing to do with it," Anne smiled mysteriously.

"Then what did?"

Her smile widened. "I surrounded him with a white light, in a white frame, and wished him love."

I groaned. "You must be putting me on."

"Try it," she said. "It works."

Lennie Weitz had already settled himself comfortably on the floor when we arrived. The young brunette behind me had a warm smile for me and the company at large.

"You don't look as tense today," she decided.

Alexander seemed to deliberately ignore the little man sprawled out at his feet. "When we go down into our levels today," he said, "we will concentrate on self-improving our minds, bodies, and health, even to eliminating headaches and general aches and pains."

As before, he suggested we first relax the eyes, then feel this relaxation moving like a wave downward through the body. We then proceeded to get into our levels, visualizing the color spectrum from Red through Violet, slowly counting down twenty-one steps, and then picturing our passive scene from nature—in my case, again the placid Pacific with its rolling surf.

As I allowed my mind to drift idly, thinking of nothing consciously, I could hear Alexander's voice dimly over my passive scene. "As I project certain phrases for your success, visualize yourself as thinking after me:

"I am now learning to develop my senses and to project my mind into any one of the levels and the depths of the different matter kingdoms. The mineral kingdom, with power of attraction, inanimate matter. The vegetable kingdom, with power to respond, plant life. The lower animal kingdom, with power of instinct. The higher animal kingdom, with the power to choose and create. The human body and mind, any one of its levels and depths."

Obviously we were now into autosuggestion, and though I saw nothing wrong with it, we were now programming ourselves, for better or worse.

"I am learning," Alexander droned, "to detect imperfections and imbalances within any one level or depth of any one kingdom."

In my role as observer and participant, I realized that we had now approached the programming area that had reshaped John Burnham and others. They had somehow reached out into the atmosphere, finding a frequency or vibratory wave which transmitted electrical energy to a misty unnamed figure in an unnamed place.

After only one day, Alexander apparently felt we were ready to be introduced to a shortcut into our levels, the finger and thumb technique.

"Now with your eyes open and holding your finger and thumb together to form a circle, pick up a book, mentally, and know that by using the finger and thumb technique, your mind will adjust instantly to your levels, and what you read will become deeply impressed on your brain cells.

"After reading, close your eyes, visualize the colors of the rainbow, enter your levels, and tell yourself: 'This information is now clearly impressed on my brain cells. From now on, all I have to do to bring back this information is to hold together my first finger and thumb of either hand to form a circle, and this information will come back as if I had just read it.'" What was done here mentally could then be done in the same way in actuality.

With lectures, Alexander advocated the same method, adding a suggestion that some speakers might find disconcerting: "To gain added concentration, continually face the lecturer and look at him eye to eye." The circling technique was similarly used in listening to the radio, watching television, or just tuning directly into one's levels.

Glancing around the room, I could see nearly everybody, including Joe, forming the finger circle and eyeballing Alexander, all but Lennie. He was snoring softly, and there was a peaceful expression on his cherubic countenance. He didn't even know he had a finger and thumb.

Alexander now passed on to specific self-help techniques. "For tension headaches, enter your levels, visualizing the rainbow. Tell your inner self that you have a headache, want to change it, and that you want to be comfortable and relaxed, your head clear and at ease. Stay in your levels for ten minutes and continue to tell yourself how you want to be. Your mind will accept these directions at your deeper levels, and on opening your eyes, your body will comply with this new pattern of thought." Reversing the colors to leave the levels, the student immediately directed his conscious mind away from the headache by doing some simple thing, such as reading a paper or phoning a friend.

The same technique was recommended for any minor ache or pain. And so, in my levels, free of the conscious mind's usual barriers, I sent this message to my sacroiliac and right shoulder, both aching from an old whiplash injury, pleased to discuss my miseries with myself, since nobody else cared about them.

Self-help steps, as enumerated by Alexander, were simple:

"One. Describe to yourself in detail how you feel and the extent of your aches and pains.

"Two. Tell yourself you do not need this discomfort, and it is unnecessary for you to suffer this way.

"Three. Stress what you need in its place and how your body, from now on, wants to feel comfortable and relaxed."

I wondered, as Alexander paused, what person thought *his* aches were minor.

He again looked around the room, his eyes again resting on the sleeping figure. With a sardonic smile and a tilt of the eyebrows, "We will now deal with a technique for staying awake for extended periods of time, when driving at night, studying for prolonged periods, working overtime, keeping an important social engagement, or"—with another look at the slumbering Lennie—"in listening to a lecture such as this."

As the class laughed, Lennie's wife, Bea, bridled indignantly. "My husband has been working twenty hours a day and he's tired."

Alexander waved his hand airly. "We've had people sleeping during the course, but never through it. But that's all right, he'll probably be the star pupil."

Again we were to enter our levels by visualizing the colors of the rainbow and saying mentally:

"One. What is wrong? I am drowsy and sleepy.

"Two. Recognize the need to change: I do not want to be drowsy or sleepy.

"Three. Tell yourself, 'I want to be wide awake, alert, and in full control of all my faculties.' "

As we came out of levels, reversing the colors of the rainbow, Alexander's eyes moved over the room. "Any questions?"

Several hands were raised.

"Yes." Alexander nodded at Joe.

"Why not use Biofeedback machines that scientifically measure your brainwaves?"

"Some teachers do, but they're still only measuring rods. We're trying to be pragmatic rather than scientific, to help people rather than experiment with them." He held up a hand. "If we can help people with a four-day course, that's more important to us than conducting tests for weeks or months. They're emphasizing the productions of brain-waves, and we're stressing self-improvement and increased awareness." His smile broadened. "If it works, why knock it?"

Joe wouldn't be put off. "How do we know it'll work?"

"After the course, you'll be given a case like everyone else. Then decide."

Another hand was raised. "Why do you say it's for only minor aches and pains?"

Alexander shrugged. "We don't want to get into medicine." He checked his watch. "One more question, and we'll break for lunch."

I found his eye. "Why don't we get in and out of our levels with the simple finger and thumb technique?"

He nodded. "It's a matter of practice, building up a habit pattern in your mind. Many graduates, who have worked at it, get into their levels by simply imagining themselves there."

Both Ralph Winters and Anne seemed pleased the way things were going. They obviously were profiting from the constant programming to relax. But like Joe, I wondered how anything that we had been doing could consistently alter the state of consciousness.

"Leave yourself open," Anne admonished.

Ralph had given the routine some thought. "As I see it, it's an autogenic process, by which we invoke the ninety percent of the mind hitherto asleep."

I laughed. "Lennie is all asleep."

Ralph looked thoughtful. "He could be getting a lot out of this."

"How do you figure?"

"In sleep, Alpha and Theta waves presumably predominate, so Lennie's in his subconscious mind practically all the time. And his autonomic processes, governed by the subconscious, are very much susceptible to suggestion."

Joe came by our table. "Can you imagine that guy telling me I'll work a case?"

"Why not give it a chance?" said Anne. "What can you lose?"

At this point, I didn't have the slightest feeling that I

could work a case, emulating John Burnham or young George Afremow. Nevertheless, I was beginning to find I could drift off into my levels with increasing rapidity.

With practice, I discovered certain images came into my mind unbidden. I was beginning to understand experiences, such as the Connecticut student's with Van Gogh, that I could never have ordinarily comprehended. Different from Yoga, the images of meditation were not immobile. They seemed to have a movement springing out of their own being. When I visualized Christ, the traditional Jesus of the Renaissance masters, a dark Latinesque figure, quickly gave way to a robust young man with reddish gold hair, blue eyes, a resolute chin and a sturdy frame. He moved in compassion and love, trailed by a company of men, some bearded, others unshaven, down the dusty road to glory. On Jesus' right was John, the dearly beloved, and on his left, a short, bearded man, whom he called Judas. "Do what you have to," he was saying to Judas.

Was this all fantasy, or had I, like the Connecticut student, tuned into a universal frequency, which philosopher Carl Jung described as a channel to every event in the annals of man?

I wasn't quite sure what the course was doing, but it was doing something. And Alexander, very much the English schoolmaster, was moving us right along. "We shall discuss survival patterns, how to form mental and physical habits for better living. PROMPT ACTION is a technique for carrying out the decisions, plans, and goals you have set for yourself, the ability to function in the present and not to procrastinate." He paused, overlooking the curled-up figure on the floor. "Enter your levels by visualizing your rainbow, then tell yourself mentally:

"One. What is wrong? Accept the fact that you habitually postpone jobs you need to do and plans for your future.

"Two. Recognize the need to change. Tell yourself you don't need to procrastinate.

"Three. Tell yourself how you want to be. Now you are going to act upon the things you need to do. There is only one time, and that is the present.

"On the Screen of the Mind, you will make a movie of yourself as the star performer. Actually see yourself being strong of mind, doing what you need to do, and doing it now. See yourself acting out positive actions in the present. Remember, as you visualize these scenes of yourself, they are deeply impressed on your brain cells."

All my life I had procrastinated, enjoying my indolence, and now Alexander was about to deprive me of one of my few pleasures. I would have blocked him out, but curiosity wouldn't be denied.

"I shall stop talking," he went on, "so that you can bring your Screen of the Mind into focus and prepare to make this movie of yourself as a person of PROMPT ACTION."

I saw myself at the typewriter, beginning a book, which I had been resisting, since it meant a total commitment for some time. My fingers literally strummed the typewriter keys, page on page, until the manuscript was completed. I saw myself happily mailing it off to the publisher, visualized the jacket and the title, and saw it in the bookstores, a best seller. How wonderful, and how unreal, for I still had the book to do.

"You have now impressed deeply on your brain cells, at this inner subjective level of the mind, an image of how you want to be, a person of PROMPT ACTION. This method can be adapted for any additional survival patterns."

Alexander faced the class leisurely, his hands in his pockets. "Many of you are wondering how all this will help your everyday life. Well, experience has shown that we are the problem, not our friends, or business associates, relatives, or even our adversaries. I know of a man who had gone from one job to another, never successful, always blaming the other fellow, until one day he found himself down to his last five dollars. He was shaving that morning, drearily contemplating his future, when he looked into the bathroom mirror and saw himself as he never had before. He stopped shaving and pointed an accusing finger into the mirror. 'You are what's wrong,' he told himself. 'Instead of gearing your efforts to other people's needs, you have thought only in terms of what would make money for you. You couldn't see what they wanted, only what you wanted, and so they turned away from you.'" He paused. "That man, with renewed enthusiasm, went out and got somebody he didn't even know to lend him the money to start a new business. Today he is a millionaire. That mirror was his Screen of the Mind."

Alexander patted his ample midsection. "In this land of plenty, a common problem is excessive weight or obesity. And since so many have this problem, we may as well use it to practice our new PROMPT ACTION technique.

"In your levels, tell yourself how you want to be, state the exact weight you wish to be. If it's a hundred and seventy or a hundred and seventeen, visualize whatever it is you want.

"Next, check out the food items that you suspect are causing an imbalance in your body. On the Screen of the Mind, place a large black 'X' over those items. See the 'X' so clearly that from now on you will not eat that particular food ever again. This is the 'Never Again' method, and from now on, whenever you see, or even think about, this particular food, see a *black 'X,'* large and clear, on it, and never again will you eat the food you have marked in this way."

For the thin or asthenic, whose problem was quite the opposite:

"To gain weight, tell yourself to be more aware of every bite of food that you take, analyze the flavor, taste it, and eat slowly, in reality enjoying and savoring every morsel that passes between your lips. Continually flash the exact image you wish to be on the Screen of the Mind, in white frame, every time you eat, think of eating, or even think about your weight.

"Let your own inner feelings choose foods best suited to your individual needs. Become aware that many foods not only lack beneficial ingredients but are harmful to your physical body. Let your inner intuitive mind lead you to choose the foods that you need. Incline more and more toward foods that are living, fresh, pure, and natural.

"Should you now, in reducing, feel, at any time, a strong urge to snack, all you need to do is to bite on a raw carrot or piece of celery, or even chew gum. This practical way of satisfying your immediate craving, through using your salivary glands, will help overcome your desire to stuff yourself at that moment."

Alexander passed to another perennial non-survival habit

problem—smoking. As a newspaperman, I had been a four-pack-a-day smoker until I kicked the habit by the simple expedient of stopping. It had been a terrible wrench, but I had not smoked for years, and found other people's smoking physically offensive. When smokers asked how I had done it, all I could say was that I had just arbitrarily quit because I did not relish being a slave to an obnoxious habit. It had reached a point where I could not pound out a news story unless I had a cigarette dangling from my lips.

Alexander's non-smoking programming was familiar, entering the levels by visualizing the colors, recognizing that smoking was a non-survival pattern, accepting the need to change, telling yourself how you wanted to be, breathing deeply of clean, fresh air, alert and in tune with life.

"Choose a day thirty days or so ahead, preferably one with special meaning for you, such as a birthday, an important anniversary, New Year's Day. Circle this day on your actual calendar and tell yourself morning and evening, in your levels, that from this day on you will never smoke again. Until the designated day comes for you to stop smoking, you may smoke as much as you like. But when this special day arrives, you stop then and there, and never smoke again. You have made a pledge, keep it, never let yourself down."

There were additional reinforcements. "See yourself on the Screen surrounded by a black frame with all the negative aspects of smoking. Consider the waste of money, the damage in making your heart beat faster as your blood vessels constrict and your glands strain to reject the poisons you have put into your body. See the dirty black smoke filling your lungs. Be aware of the acrid smell of stale tobacco on your skin as you perspire, and on your clothes, which reek with the same dank smell.

"Now see yourself in a white frame. Your lungs are pink and smooth and healthy, sending vitalizing oxygen through your bloodstream to your entire body. Your home is brighter and cleaner, free of cigarette smells and stains. Your body is clean, pure, vital."

Smoking was a difficult habit to stop. The smoker constantly deluded himself that he could quit whenever necessary for his health.

"Every day visualize the circle date on the calendar, as your Never Again date, so as to get your body and brain cells to conform to this new pattern of being able to breathe freely and deeply of life-giving oxygen. When you feel the urge to smoke, take a deep breath three times, and this will help to remove the craving. Just three long, deep breaths, and the desire to smoke will pass."

I remembered now, as Alexander spoke, that I had reinforced my own resolve to stop smoking by taking a swallow of water whenever I wanted a cigarette. In a way, I had programmed myself, and what made it additionally easier, I now recalled, was a highly visual experience in which, at four in the morning, with all shops, bars, and drugstores closed, I had begged a cigarette from a street bum, who had just put the touch on me. I could almost smell that twisted bit of weed that the moocher had extricated with grimy hand from a dirty pocket. And I had taken it gratefully, greedily inhaling each glob of smoke as if it were my last.

As I now recognized the influencing visualization of my real-life experience, I could dimly hear Alexander discussing how children could be programmed long before they would normally reach for their first cigarette.

"You may indoctrinate them not to smoke when they are very young children, even babies, when they are asleep." A ripple of laughter raced through the room, but Lennie sweetly slept through it. "Tell them that when they get older they will not smoke. Even if they don't understand at the outer conscious level, they will pick up this information at the inner subjective level of the mind, and you will find that when they grow up they will not smoke."

We were now ready to leave our levels, with the reverse color sequence.

I saw Red and opened my eyes. I turned my head slowly. The girl behind me was smiling benevolently. "You don't seem as tense as you did," she said, touching me on the shoulder.

It was time for a break. "When we get back," said Alexander, "you will learn how to put your mind to good use while your physical body rests and sleeps."

Lennie yawned and rubbed his eyes. "What time is it?" he asked.

Chapter 5

The Dream World

Miracles were only that which we did not understand. Before Faraday, electric power was a fantasy; before the Wright brothers, only birds could fly; Abraham Lincoln struck a phosphorus match and wondered what the next miracle would be. Somewhere in nature there were frequencies into which gifted man could direct his thoughts and energies, tuning into the life around him and receiving similar impulses in return. He could perform these wonders in the waking state, when his conscious mind was laid to rest through meditation. In sleep, with his Beta mind supplanted by the slower, deeper brainwave rhythms of Alpha-Theta, he could presumably do more.

Now Alexander was telling us about the water technique as a simple way of getting the sleeping, dreaming mind to help us. This was a trigger devise, causing the mind to search for and find solutions to projects—never problems, a negative concept—when fast asleep.

We were already in our levels, inducted in the usual way, and Alexander was programming us to look for connections between our dreams and events normally overlooked, like a phone call, a chance meeting, a letter, anything that might turn our lives around if recognized and acted upon.

"You will go through an actual cycle, using a project that you have in mind, a project whose outcome is as yet unknown. Select a project which seems to be causing you concern and which you would like to solve at this time.

"I shall count from one to three, and at the count of three, you will project yourself to your home and see yourself in bed, preparing to go to sleep, with a glass of water by your bedside.

"Just before you go off to sleep, close your eyes, turn them slightly upward, and say to yourself mentally:

" 'This is all I have to do to find the solution to the project I have in mind.' Then drink half the water and rest your thoughts of finding a solution to your project. Enter a deep, sound sleep. In the morning, when you awaken, close your eyes again, and again turn them slightly upward [a way of inviting Alpha]. While drinking the remaining half of the water in the glass, repeat to yourself mentally:

" 'This is all I have to do to find the solution to the project I have in mind.'

"The solution to your project will either come in the form of a dream during the night, which you will understand and which will help you solve your project or it will be in your thoughts when you awaken in the morning, or it may come during the following day as a flash of insight or an intuitive impression which will lead you to a perfect solution of your project.

"Since the solution may come in ways you least expect, be especially attentive for the special significance of ordinary events and means of communication. You will find that the solution to your project will come in due course. This psychological trigger device will cause your mind to search for and find solutions to projects when you are asleep."

To establish that sleep suggestion worked, Alexander now discussed a simple technique for waking up at a desired time. I had practiced this during Yoga-training and could retire with the suggestion that I be up at seven or seven-fifteen, or seven-o-two, and it would work. Once the clock said six-thirty, but it had run down during the night, and the true time was the programmed seven-o-two. The suggestion was merely planted during the meditation period that followed the physical exercises and reinforced before bedtime.

Alexander called the technique the mental alarm clock.

"When you are in bed and ready to go to sleep, enter your levels. Then tell yourself mentally:

" 'I want to wake up at such-and-such a time.' At the

same time, see your mental alarm clock clearly in your mind and see yourself moving the hands of this clock to the exact time you want to wake up. Say to yourself, 'This is the time I want to wake up. This is the time I am going to wake up.'

"Then go to sleep while in your levels. You will then wake up in perfect health, feeling revitalized and refreshed, and in tune with life, at the exact time you desired."

Sleep induction was a perfectly natural next step.

I had concluded that being in my levels was tantamount to having turned off my conscious mind. Since nature abhors a vacuum, the subconscious state very naturally introduced itself as the intellectual mind receded. Sleep had always been a bit of a problem, and I looked forward, to Alexander's announcement that he was about to confer the instant boon of slumber on insomniacs. "For the problem sleeper, this is a method," said Alexander, "of entering normal sleep without the use of pills or drugs of any kind.

"In bed, and ready for sleep, close your eyes and visualize mentally a blackboard and yourself standing before it with chalk in one hand and an eraser in the other. Now draw a large circle on your mental blackboard. Next, write the number 100 inside the circle, just touching the circle, careful to keep the number 100 completely within the circle. Now slowly erase the number 100, working from the center toward the circumference of the circle, careful not to erase the circle itself.

"Then write the word SLEEP, large and clear, in a flowing hand, just outside and to the right of the circle. Now repeat the process with the descending numbers 99, 98, 97, etc., remembering to trace over the word SLEEP each time. Continue with these descending numbers and I will stop talking to you for a while."

I had reached 89, but I still wasn't sleepy, when Alexander resumed.

"Relax, take a deep breath and relax. Should you happen to wake up during the night, or before the time you wish to wake up, all you have to do is to rearrange your pillow and you will go directly to sleep.

"Every time you use sleep induction in this manner, you

will enter normal, natural sleep, anytime, anywhere, simply with the proper use of your mind."

We left our levels the usual way, visualizing the reverse flow of the rainbow.

I opened my eyes to find Alexander looking at the sleeping Lennie in annoyance.

"The supreme test of this course," he said, "would be to keep that man awake."

As we all laughed, Lennie's wife loyally came to his support. "The test should be whether he gets anything out of his sleep."

My mind had wandered restlessly, bored by the tedium of the countdown. Obviously Alexander was programming his students with suggestions, repeated for reinforcement, but he did not appear to exercise the absolute controls of the hypnotist. In no way were our wills externally controlled. I was free, as were the others, to accept what I wanted of his suggestions and make them self-regulating controls. The authority appeared to remain in my hands. I had to tell myself that something was going to work, I had to be expectant and open, and not unless I kept visualizing the suggestions at home, creating a new brainwave pattern, would there be any lasting effect. Given this technique, we still had to program ourselves to cut through mental blocks and attain the critical self-analysis and self-knowledge that would, hopefully, illuminate the rest of our days.

Alexander's suggestions, at all times, were ostensibly constructive—to be more creative, productive, and healthy, with a zest for living. I wasn't sure how this would work. I had listened all my life to admonitions from parent figures, teachers, clergy, physicians, friends. We all knew it was better to think positively than negatively. Nobody wanted to shoulder other people's problems. When we laughed, the world laughed with us; crying, we cried alone.

There was something very specific about Alexander's programming. I had programmed myself to wake at a certain time, but not with a technique I could repeat at will. I had somehow gotten into my subconscious mind through Yogic breathing and meditation, but without a step-by-step technique, I had no assurance of repeating the desired result.

Alexander provided the steps, giving confidence of the outcome. Once again, in our levels, he outlined the steps for showing the student how to use more of his mind on a daily basis.

Step One was a sequel to the dream programming:

"On awakening, immediately write down anything you may recall from your sleep during the night, such as a dream—what it was and what its significance seems to be. Your recollection may seem unimportant at first, but with practice, you will bring more of value into your waking state. This information may actually produce solutions to projects that you set your mind to work on while your body is asleep. Or they may fill in information essential for you at this time, or spark intuitive flashes that may lead to something significant during the day.

"Keep a writing pad by your bedside and write down whatever comes at once, together with what you intend to do during the coming day. Put what seems most important at the top of your list, no matter how difficult it appears. The sense of accomplishment from successfully carrying out the large tasks makes the smaller ones easier to do.

"Allocate reasonable time for what you need to do. Set yourself a schedule, dividing up the available time to the best advantage for the goals you set yourself for that day. Don't overload yourself, make sure the plans you do make are fulfilled to the best of your ability."

We were about to program ourselves. "Go through the list, item by item, stating exactly what you need to do. Bring the Screen of the Mind into focus and make a movie of yourself as the star performer, acting out the jobs you have set for yourself. See yourself accomplishing each job, one by one. See yourself confident and courageous, decisive and enthusiastic, happy and healthy, honest and loving.

"As you act out these tasks in this manner, mentally they will become so impressed on your brain cells that later that day your body will accomplish these tasks with ease, at the outer physical level. Stay in your levels ten to fifteen minutes, setting your goals in the manner just described."

I had no intention of doing anything to encourage my dreams. I had enough to do all day without troubling about what I was thinking during the night. If needed, this was still another indication that the instructor wielded no magic spell over his class.

However, I did join in the planning cycle. At the count of three, already in my levels, I projected myself on the Screen of the Mind and visualized myself interviewing people in the class about their reactions, and I programmed myself to remember everything Alexander had said, so that I could readily explain it to anybody who might be interested.

Step Two appeared to implement Step One.

"During the day, physically act out to the best of your ability that which you have decided and planned to do. Taking these jobs in the proper order, one by one, act out each task until it becomes an actuality, just as you planned in the movie projected on the Screen of the Mind. Be aware of an inspired level of mind that will help you accomplish what you need to do. Be especially attentive to ordinary events and communication that may provide leads on how to effectively bring your plans to fruition."

Reinforcement could be helpful!

"The middle of the day (say, just after lunch) go to your levels by visualizing the colors of the rainbow. Stay in your levels for some ten minutes to gain extra guidance, peace of mind, and physical rest, so you will be able to function more effectively for the remainder of the day. Recharging your batteries, you will have an even clearer mind and gain physical energy to do whatever you have to do.

"Also use the finger and thumb technique to adjust quickly to the inner subjective level for greater mind power whenever needed. Anytime you have an impulse that you should do anything, make a notation of it and later record this information on your bedside pad for use in making plans for the next day. By continual effort, your plans are bound to materialize. Let each accomplishment become one more brick in the road to health, wealth, and happiness."

I couldn't help thinking, as I sat, detached, observing Alexander's technique, of the poor farmer advised in a vision of a pot of gold buried in his acreage. Every morning he got up, bright and early, programmed to dig in a different section of his neglected forty acres. In a week, he had dug up the whole place without finding gold. With the land all plowed up, he decided he might as well scatter some seed on it. In the fall, he had a bumper crop, paid off the mortgage, made needed repairs, and had money to spare. He had indeed taken treasure out of the land.

And so, if one pushed enough, in the right direction, with the proper enthusiasm, it was quite possible he would meet success halfway. I found myself already doing some of the things Alexander suggested. Every morning, I mentally planned my workday, promising myself a walk on the beach after writing five pages and a hot tub after ten pages. Before addressing the typewriter, I got the most unpleasant chores out of the way first, so they wouldn't cloud my day.

Over my reverie, Alexander was into Step Three:

"Before going to sleep for the night, visualize yourself into your levels and review the day for ten minutes. Praise yourself where you have successfully achieved a goal that you had set for yourself that day. This helps to make deeper impressions on your brain cells, so that your achievements become permanent. Next, reappraise the failures in bringing into being what you had intended to do. Check out and see what went wrong. Tell your mind this is not what you want, then tell your mind, once again, what you need to do.

"Remember your mind never goes to sleep—it functions twenty-four hours a day. So just before going to sleep, use the glass-of-water technique to help you to find out about anything that happened during the past day that you didn't understand, or to solve any project, large or small, to which you need a solution to help you be more effective the following day.

"Set the hands of your mental alarm clock to the exact time you want to awaken. Then go to sleep, still in your levels, knowing that you will wake up at the exact time you desired.

"If you wish to make certain that you go to sleep immediately after you have reviewed the past day, you may use the sleep-induction technique on the Screen of the

Mind, and so count yourself down into a deep, peaceful, and profitable night's sleep."

And so we passed on to Step Four:

"When your body is physically asleep, know that your mind is constantly in action. Be assured that your mind is working according to the directions you gave it prior to going to sleep. Have confidence that solutions are being found in the storehouse of your own memory banks, or are being given to you from the Universal Mind. On awakening, you will receive information to help you become a balanced and successful person."

As I prepared to stir out of my levels, I hazily heard Alexander's final injunction: "Go and serve your fellow man with love in your daily life and be a light to the world."

I put a white light around myself and went through the reverse sequence of the rainbow. I sat up, still in the half-world of my own reverie, feeling incredibly refreshed, with a surprising sense of kinship for my fellows. I even saw Joe as a poor errant soul, trying lucklessly to get in step. I was not alone. Linda Lockwood, Eve Bruce, Anne Francis, and the others appeared to be radiating a new inner glow. The face of the sweet young thing behind me shone with an almost ethereal loveliness.

"You still seem tense," she said softly. "Would you like me to massage your shoulders?"

Chapter 6

The Workshop

In the imaginary Workshop, in our levels, we would begin applying the wonders of our expanding intelligence. Here we would solve cases, tune into the universe, see into other people's hearts and minds, and more importantly, into our own.

"What a crock," said Joe with a singular lack of imagination.

"Joe," I said, "why don't you get your money back?"

He gave me an abrasive look. "You don't think the man would?"

"I think he'd be glad to. Your vibrations are rocking the boat."

He sniffed scornfully. "Some boat."

We had been trapped at the same table over our pre-class coffee.

"What about this Universal Mind that's going to make us all so smart?"

"You've got to leave yourself open," said I, trying to program love and patience, "and be expectant."

He gave me a scrutinizing look. "Do you honestly believe these idiots will be able to tune into something as nebulous as the Universal Mind?"

"According to the mystic Edgar Cayce, and to Doctor Carl Gustav Jung, one of the great minds of our time, the Universal Mind contains a record of everything that has happened and is going to happen."

"And you believe that?" He swallowed the last of his coffee.

I found my new patience wearing thin. "You can limit the world to your own horizons, if you like."

67

He trailed after me into the classroom. I looked around the room, nodding at Ernie Dade, the Hollywood agent, who was floating on air from the changes already taking place after only two days. "I feel relaxed and liberated," he told me, "as if I could do anything, or influence anybody, so long as it was for good."

"Just don't try walking on water," I cautioned.

I felt, almost insensibly, a weaving together of minds, as if all in the room were being mentally or spiritually joined by their efforts to project an extending awareness.

My eyes almost mechanically turned to little Lennie. He needed no programming. He was already curled up on the floor, with a blanket tucked to his chin, breathing evenly.

Alexander repeated the usual three cycles to put us in our levels, visualizing the colors, counting down and viewing the nature scene. However, many in the class, like Ralph Winters and Linda Lockwood, were already into their levels before they reached the end of the rainbow.

They were eager to mentally construct the Workshop, which was to be the scene of their future development. "Creating a Workshop serves the dual purpose of not only developing the imagination," said Alexander, "but of providing the means to work on various projects.

"I shall count from twelve to one, and as I do so, see yourself on the count of one entering this creative, imaginative, inspired Workshop level. Now I shall count from one to three, and by the time I reach three, you will have created your Workshop."

As we poised at the door of our Workshops, Alexander entered his own Workshop, so that communication between teacher and student would be at a peak level. "Communication is always more direct," he explained, "when there is an energy exchange on the same plateau of the mind.

"One. Mentally using hands, lay the foundations and the floor. Then bring into being and create the walls, and finally the ceiling. Make the Workshop what size you like, and the shape and design you desire. Use materials that appeal to you, in creating this room, floor, walls, and ceiling.

"Two. You are both the architect and the builder. Pay attention to details and create your Workshop exactly as you want it to be.

"Three. If you want to add, change, or remodel, you may do so anytime you are in your Workshop level. You are now ready to furnish your Workshop. I will mention a few things you may wish to put into the Workshop, but you can add or subtract anything you like. It is your Workshop, to do what you want with it."

I had visualized as a Workshop the city room of a newspaper where I had worked for years, and had conveniently located it on a bluff of the Pacific rather than in dismal, dreary, depressing New York City.

"You would probably first install a chair and table. The chair should be comfortable and to your liking, since you will often sit in this chair. It is good to have a panel built into an arm of the chair to control lighting, etc. The table should be circular and designed to be used for conferences.

"You may need a telephone. A large, executive type, with several buttons to push to get various lines directly.

"Clock and calendar. Capable of going backward or forward in time either to review the past and look into what made a certain situation a failure or a success or to project into the future to plan total success.

"Files and reference books. These files will contain financial records, analyses of different situations, research reports, and business proposals covering the past, present, future. These reference books should be encyclopedic, where the exact information can be found.

"Television screen and visual aids. This screen may be used in conjunction with your telephone so that you can lock onto the actual person with whom you are trying to communicate. The visual aids may be either still or moving pictures, and may even be three-dimensional. Instruments and appliances may cover any conceivable need, from music to lighting, refrigeration and heating.

"Platform and Screen. These are to be placed at the far end of your Workshop, opposite your chair. Make the platform small, yet large enough to place a person on it. You may carpet it if you wish. The Screen is directly behind the platform. You may use this from now on as the

Screen of the Mind when you are in your Workshop. Put some overhead lights on the ceiling to shine on the platform and illuminate the Screen. These lights should be controlled by switches on the arm of your chair, for you are the master of your Workshop.

"Elevator. Just to the right of your platform create an elevator and make it in such a way that the door of this elevator slides down into the floor. This elevator is used to bring anything that you may need from another dimension. Place the door control of this elevator on the arm of your chair."

I mentally put into my Workshop everything Alexander suggested, and more—an oblong table, with a large center slot for myself, such as that used by copy editors; a walkie-talkie with which I could communicate with anybody I wanted; and an automatic typewriter, which typed by itself. I had a number of pictures on the wall: Jesus, David, Moses, Michelangelo, Leonardo, Lincoln, Gandhi, Edison, Einstein. My Workshop was well-stocked with miracle workers, and all I could hope was that some of this magic would rub off.

During the coffee break, Anne Francis' eyes were bright with expectancy. "This course is an actor's delight," she said. "In your Workshop, you can get to be the producer, director, writer, and star, then put yourself on your Screen of the Mind and toss the script to the winds."

Ralph Winters, used to working with artistic people, was enthusiastic over the possibilities. "It should stimulate creative people and wake up others."

Alexander had promised to introduce two imaginary assistants into our Workshops, to help us with our problems—or projects. They were to be our servants, not masters, and of our own choosing, involuntary or deliberate. "They may just materialize without you consciously doing anything about it," Alexander said.

"Who will you pick?" I asked Anne.

"I'm not going to let anybody know who's helping me. They might steal them away."

I saw Joe in the distance and averted my gaze, but he stopped by anyway to confide in a mock whisper, "I'm making Alexander my assistant. He seems to know everything."

As before, we visualized ourselves into our levels with the rainbow and reinforced with the countdown from twenty-one, feeling ourselves deeper and deeper within.

"To bring into being your two assistants, return to your creative, imaginative Workshop level. Review everything you have created so far. Check out the floor, walls, and ceiling, then the furnishings and equipment. Make any changes you wish."

He mentioned each object in turn, adding a few words of description. "You have now checked out your entire Workshop. Next, take a seat behind your table and look in the direction of your elevator door—and be prepared to bring in your assistants."

There were to be two, male and female. They were to be real or imaginary, from this lifetime or whatever. "First of all, you will bring into being your male assistant. This man, at this moment, is behind the sliding door in your elevator. [His face vaguely took form in my mind for the first time.] Now use the control on the arm of your chair to cause the door of your elevator to move slightly downward.

"Bring the door down just a little way. Notice the color of his hair, the exact shade. Observe the thickness, and whether it's long or short. Is his hair combed and in place, or is it disarranged?"

As the elevator door gradually slid down, more and more of the face became visible. "Now see his forehead. See the actual skin on his forehead and look at it closely. Are there any lines or wrinkles on his forehead, or is the skin smooth and firm?"

I had picked an assistant out of real life, but oddly, his features changed as I examined him. He was two-faced.

"Pause for a few moments," Alexander droned, "to make a thorough study of your male assistant. Observe his face in detail and look into his eyes."

The body was to gradually emerge. "Keep your hand on the control switch on the arm of your chair, to keep the door moving down slowly, exposing the body a little at a time. You now have a good idea of what he looks like."

We had created a Frankenstein, whether a modified version of somebody we knew, a real-life psychic in my case, or pure invention, out of a memory pattern newly woven from some hitherto unused portion of the mind.

The personality was also crystallizing. "He is dynamic and alive as he walks into your Workshop. Greet him and mentally ask his name. As you talk to him, become aware of his presence and realize he is a real person, and that he is with you in your Workshop. Walk around your Workshop with him and show him what you have put in and how it works. Ask him to sit next to you, or stand nearby, always there, just to your right, ready to help you anytime you need him."

I had no great plans for my assistant. But the exercises in visualization had been edifying. I now saw an imagined individual so clearly that I could almost reach out and touch him. If my assistant never lifted a finger, I had still gained creatively from the experience.

For the female assistant, the procedure was repeated. I found myself choosing an old lady in her nineties, a saintly figure who had helped countless people with her counsel.

"These assistants," said Alexander, "can assist, instruct, guide, and counsel you at all levels, but you yourselves are always in charge and actually do the work. They are there only in an advisory capacity."

He paused. "Now, thank your assistants for being with you and tell them you look forward to being with them again the next time you enter the Workshop."

With the reverse sequence of the rainbow, we were back in the room, stretching, yawning, rubbing our eyes, and looking around at one another, half-expectantly. I sensed a feeling of relaxation and peace, a pervasive warmth that seemed to fill the room. Anne, Ralph, Linda, Eve, were all smiling; Suzie, behind me, had a sparkle in her eyes; even Lennie was awake and beaming. I looked about covertly for Joe. He was scowling and I could see his lips curl disdainfully. "What a crock."

I sighed, knowing the world was full of Joes.

As we filed out for the break, I could hear students eagerly discussing their assistants.

"Mine," said one, "is a Tibetan monk, who keeps the Akashic record, an account of everything that has ever happened on this earth plane."

"And mine," said another, "is Albert Einstein. Who could know more than he?"

It all seemed to be in fun, and then I saw a faint frown on Ralph's brow. Just a step behind us, a student had proclaimed, in a voice perhaps louder than he intended, "Jesus is my assistant."

I shuddered to think who his female assistant might be, and moved off quickly.

Ralph looked musingly at his coffee. "This assistant thing could be a bit of an ego trip."

"I don't see why we can't do it ourselves if there's anything to this Alpha thinking."

Ralph gulped his coffee. "I think I'll dispense with assistants."

I mentioned my qualms to Alexander.

His face took on a speculative look. "Unless your assistants come to you on a subconscious level, with no calculation by your conscious mind, they won't be of any real use."

"I picked mine consciously."

He shook his head. "And that is why you rejected them; they didn't fit into your deeper level of thinking. Actually the assistants are personifications of your subconscious mind, a psychological trigger device to help you accept your new awareness."

"And did your assistants come to you unbidden?"

He nodded. "Yes, one was a Tibetan lama."

I thought of the many dangers inherent in a wide-open subconscious. Entities, which could be capricious earthbound spirits, were a potential problem. "Suppose some malignant entity were to take you over in the guise of an assistant?"

Alexander surprised me by nodding solemnly. "It happens sometimes, but a teacher should be able to spot it. In a way, since the entity reflects a hidden state of mind, it is better revealed than concealed."

I was onto more than I had bargained for. "But how would you spot these cases?"

"A few students have turned up animals as assistants, apparently symbolizing a lurking force for evil. It should be summarily rejected as that person is locked into a negative state." He could recall only one such case among his thousands of students.

"One young woman brought up an assistant in the form of a serpent. I promptly told her that she didn't need anything like this, and that she should go into her levels and dismiss him." Allegorically, of course, this was base temptation.

In Manchester, England, a student had approached Alexander trembling from head to foot, in a cold sweat. He seemed to have seen a ghost. "I felt he was possessed, and in front of the class, I took him down to his levels and ordered the entity out of him."

"And how did you do that?" I asked perfunctorily, having never really believed in demons.

Alexander's face became grave. "I told him, 'This power will leave your body and mind. It has nothing to do with you now, and it will be replaced by a higher consciousness that will dispel all evil within you. Open your Workshop door, and two true assistants will come in and take its place.' "

Later he discovered the student had been a medium for a spiritualist group and was habitually open to entities. "It would never happen with the ordinary human being."

To expand our senses, developing our Alpha imagery, we now projected our minds into various forms of matter: metal, stone, wood, fruit. Everett held up a small block of lead which we visually transferred into our Workshops. It was smooth and cold, with the dank touch of heavy metal. "Bring the block slowly to your forehead until it actually touches the skin," he said. "And then, with a snap of the fingers, effect a change of size so that you can visually crawl into the block of lead and observe it with all five senses." It was no task at all to make a house of lead. The procedure was repeated with an orange, a piece of wood, a rough stone—and each time the reaction was sharper and clearer. With the orange, I could practically taste the juice.

Continuing the sense-expanding program, Alexander now took us on a visual tour of nature. In communing with the four seasons, would I feel mystically merged in the secret scheme of ever-renewing life?

"Walk over to your calendar," Alexander was saying, "and set it for January, the season of winter. Next, walk to the other end of your Workshop, just to the left of your Screen. Open a door and see the peaceful countryside set out before you. The rolling hills are blanketed with snow. The trees, bushes, and all the varied vegetation are lying dormant beneath a covering of white. Notice how the stream and ponds are iced over. Now walk out into the snow, feel it crunching under your feet, stoop down and pick up some snow, and rub it between your fingers. Feel the delicate crystals melt in your hands."

I could almost feel my fingers tingling with the cold, growing first red and then white. "Make a snowball if you like, and roll it along the ground. The ice on the stream and ponds reflects the silence and the peacefulness of this wintry landscape. Notice the trees and how the naked branches stand out against the skyline. Drink in the quietude of this white crystalline purity, hear the very silence, feel the forces of nature as they rest in this dormant winter state."

We moved on to spring. "The snow has all melted, and wherever you look, you see a light shade of green. Everything looks clean and fresh. The sap is rising in the trees, the buds are opening, there are beautiful blossoms in delicate shades of pink and white. Pick a blossom, examine it closely, and feel how delicate it is. Smell the blossom, become aware of its beautiful fragrance. [I could almost taste the lilacs.]

"Use all your senses to communicate with nature. Hear the birds singing, smell the fragrance in the air, savor all the beauties of spring, and feel stirred by the awakening forces around you."

Alexander continued into summer and July.

"The trees and the vegetation are now darker green. The grass is longer and more luxuriant, the leaves and branches fuller and thicker. See the butterflies flitting by, notice the exquisite colors and delicate form of their wings. Hear the bees and watch them making their rounds, pollinating the flowers. The flowers are in full bloom, so bend down and feel the softness of the petals, note the intensity and softness of the colors. Smell it, how does the fragrance of this flower seem to you? Listen to the birds and the sounds of animal life."

"Now pause a moment and sit down under a tree in the shade. Pick up a blade of grass and put it in your mouth and taste the fullness of summer. Lean back against a tree and view the overall scene. Look at the horses and cattle in the distance, swishing their tails to keep the flies off. It is hot, and many of the animals, like yourself, have sought refuge in the shade. There is a heaviness in the air. Be aware of both the visible and the invisible stirrings within the vegetable and lower animal kingdoms. Nature has reached her peak. Feel the radiance and joy of this time, the season of summer."

In October, nature reached her fulfillment.

"The trees are clothed in shades of red, gold, and orange, the grass streaked with grayish brown and covered with leaves. This is the time of harvest, the berries, fruits, and nuts are ripe and ready to pick. Pick a nut or berry and examine it closely. Taste it, and savor it, and enjoy the fruits of autumn.

"These changing seasons have been deeply impressed on your brain cells, so that you will be able to move through time or space with ease anytime you desire."

I had now been inside an orange, a hunk of lead, a piece of wood, and the four seasons.

"Next," said Alexander, "you will learn to make further points of reference, this time in the physical body of a human being.

"Concentrate first on the top of your head, move down to your forehead, the eyes, cheeks, jaw, neck, and shoulders. Feel your lungs breathing rhythmically, your heart beating in a normal and natural way. Next, moving slowly down the body, become aware of each part of your body, all the way down to the feet.

"Become aware of your mind in the soles of your feet, gradually pull it up to your knees, then your waist, chest, neck, and head. You are now aware only of your head. Gather together all your awareness [I could hear Lennie

76

gently snoring] into the brain area, then place your total awareness in suspension in space over your head."

"I am able," I repeated mentally after Alexander, "to develop my awareness and to project my mind to any place on this earth, and will know what is going on, should this be helpful to mankind."

It was with a sense of relief that I found myself back in the comforting drabness of the classroom. As I looked around, everybody seemed friendlier and more open, with the exception of the incorrigible Joe. We were all eyeing each other closely, looking for changes that might mirror our own transformation. Lennie was apparently more relaxed than ever, falling off to sleep quicker and sleeping sounder. His wife's cheeks appeared to glow with a new vitality.

On this fourth and final day, nearly all had misgivings about the upcoming test cases. Accordingly, Alexander guided us into our levels for a brush-up tour of a human body.

"See the form and shape of a friend. See this person three-dimensioned, clearly standing there."

I picked out a young lady three thousand miles away.

"Ask this person to move around, facing in different directions, alive and real, walking around and smiling."

Mentally I examined the girl's skin, bones, nerves, and muscles. My subject was well-muscled for a girl. She played tennis, swam, danced, and appeared in good shape. Yet I noticed her lungs were dark and sooty. And then I remembered she was a chain-smoker.

We invoked the image of still another friend and put his head on. I picked a young man who had once pledged me undying gratitude. He was a professional psychic, whom I had helped.

"Pick up his head and place it over yours, as you would a large hat," said Alexander. "Let it slip over your head, right down to your shoulders. Try to sense through this person's brain what he feels and thinks. Is he loving and kind, sad or upset, even hateful and angry? Try to grasp this person's basic mood. It may not be at all what you would expect."

My friend had always appeared properly appreciative.

Yet, now, his lips were a thin, hard line and his eyes pinpoints of resentment.

"How," asked Alexander, "does this person feel about life, money, and friends?" I suddenly saw him as acquisitive and vain, brushing back a lock of his hair while stealing a glimpse at the mirror.

"Now that you have made contact with your friend, ask if there is anything he would like to tell you."

I saw angry words framed on the mean little mouth. "Other people pay for my advice. They look up to me, just as I look down at you. I don't need you anymore."

"Talk to your friend mentally, making suggestions and giving advice at this inner level. Visualize perfect end results, flashing this result on the Screen of the Mind in a white frame."

I calmly rejected Alexander's suggestion. So, clearly, I was not being hypnotized. Actually my own control seemed to be increasing. If there was any hypnosis, it was autogenic, self-accepted and self-generated.

"Call on Higher Intelligence," said Alexander, "to produce the desired pattern of behavior for this person. Feel within you peace, strength, love, then project this pattern to the person you wish to help. With Higher Intelligence as a guide, only good can come from projecting in this way."

He paused for a few moments.

"Take this person's head off and put him back, mentally, on the platform. Thank him for being cooperative and assure him that the information you received will be kept confidential."

I had heard enough to jog my memory and tell me I had the right head on.

Many were facing their test cases with trepidation. Ralph Winters seemed the coolest of all. "At least," he said, "we had a pleasant four days together."

Lennie had risen for lunch, and passed us with a smile.

"He hasn't done anything but rest," somebody said caustically.

Ralph disagreed. "He's made a major contribution. He's given us something to be amused about, and, more significantly, if he does well, it means that the subconscious mind actually operates independent of the conscious faculties."

Alexander gave us our final instructions in our levels. "Be calm, still, and at peace as you mentally project yourself into your passive scene from nature. Think positively, not only for your own benefit but to help other people and serve mankind.

"In a few minutes, you will project your mind into the body and mind of another person and detect any imperfections. The moderator will guide you into your Workshop level, then give you what information you need to work your case. Just lock onto the Screen of the Mind, put the person in a white frame, and know that you will succeed. Take the impressions that come to mind first. Use your abilities wisely, and your power will increase. Always tell yourself after working a case that a sense of peace will come over you and your body will be in perfect health. Now visualize the colors in reverse sequence to bring yourself back to the conscious level." He paused. "When you open your eyes, you will be wide awake, feeling revitalized and in tune with life. Good luck."

Chapter 7

Tested

Anne Francis turned to me nervously. "I know they'll call on me first. And I just know I'm going to make a fool of myself. I can't remember a thing."

"It'll come back," I said, reassuring myself in the same breath.

I looked around the room. The handful of graduates, who had come down from San Francisco, were sifting through slips of paper with our test cases.

"I should be joining them," said Suzie, the beautiful teenager who sat behind me.

"You?" I said incredulously.

"Oh, yes," she said nonchalantly. "I'm a graduate. That's how I knew you were so tense. I put your head on my shoulders that first day, and it almost gave me a headache." She smiled. "But you're better now; relaxing in your levels does it."

"So you think it proper to look into another person's head?"

"Of course, if you intend to help them."

"And if you plan to do just the opposite?"

This thought had apparently never struck her. "Alexander says that the power fails if you try to do anything but good with it."

She got up and sauntered off as Alexander asked the moderators to step forward.

I noticed Joe in a back row, waving his hands and speaking loudly. Linda Lockwood and Eve Bruce seemed composed, almost expectant, and Ralph Winters appeared confident.

Little Lennie was rubbing his eyes, looking about sleepily, but making a visible effort to get to his feet.

I didn't know whom to feel sorrier for, Lennie or the graduate who had to give him his case.

Alexander's voice recalled me to the present. "Anne Francis," he said with a nod for the actress, "will work the first case."

Anne gave me a disgusted look. "See!"

She moved to the front of the room. Her case was a fifty-year-old man. That was all the information she was given. She looked about helplessly for a moment; then Alexander's voice came in pleasantly, instructing her to go to her levels as before, relax, and let the image form on the Screen of her Mind.

"It should be easy for an actor to get into somebody else's head," he said. "They do it all the time."

The moderator sat next to Anne, with a slip of paper listing the problem. "We'll start with the head; do you see anything there?"

She shook her head.

Next came the face, the nose, mouth, throat, and still nothing. Then the shoulders, chest, abdomen, with Anne's voice faltering a little as nothing seemed to be coming through.

"I see this person in a home with yellow drapes," she said uncertainly. "Could that be right?"

The moderator shrugged. "It could be, but it's not on the slip. We can check that later."

Thus far, Anne's performance seemed to justify her fears. The inventory on a descending level had now reached the legs, and I was beginning to empathize, not with the the unknown subject but with my friend and fellow student.

As I threw her my moral support, I noticed the beginning of an uncertain frown. She had zeroed into something on her own, and it was obviously something unusual.

The moderator leaned forward encouragingly. "Tell us what you see, however fantastic and unbelievable it may seem."

Anne's voice was stronger now. "I see this leg, it's withered, and I see steel around it. It's a brace."

The moderator checked his slip. "That's right, this person has a steel brace on his leg."

Anne's eyes had been closed, helping her to visualize. She now opened them wide and looked around with an expression of surprised gratification. "I thought for a while I might be the class dunce."

There was one error. Anne had pictured the right leg instead of the left, and Alexander, who was familiar with the case, pointed out that she had not reversed her image on the Screen, a customary mistake with novices.

"Distribute yourselves around the room, and a graduate will give each of you a case," Alexander announced pleasantly. "Expect to be successful, and you will be. Don't give substance to negative suggestions."

My case had been presented by agent Ernie Dade's wife, Grace, a schoolteacher. All I was given was a ten-year-old boy; no address, no name, no anything. I suspected he had an illness or malfunction of some sort or he wouldn't have become a case. But that was my only clue.

A number of people had formed a circle around me, including Grace and the precocious Suzie.

"Just go through the color cycle," the moderator was saying, "and the twenty-one countdown, visualize your passive scene from nature, and then enter your Workshop to the count of twelve. Relax and remember that it will be very easy for you to put this person on the Screen of the Mind. If you need your assistants, they will always be available."

I went through the cycles methodically, visualized the familiar surf, and slipped into my Workshop. There was nobody there but me and the unnamed presence I was to conjure on the Screen in my imaginary room. I had long before dismissed my assistants.

"In your levels, looking at your Screen," the moderator said, "examine the subject's scalp, hair, and forehead, the skin texture, and then the interior of the head, the brain, its network of nerves and blood vessels."

My eyes closed, passing over a nebulous gray mass, but at the same time altogether healthy.

"Do you find anything wrong there?"

I shook my head.

"Now the ears and the eyebrows. And the eyes. Look

at the eyes closely. What do you see about the eyes? Is there anything about the eyes?" The moderator's voice was insistent.

So there was something wrong with the eyes. What could it be? The possibilities were virtually endless, and my only knowledge of eyes had come from casual conversations with ophthalmologists while being examined for glasses.

I didn't see in shades of pink or black, I didn't know if it was nerves, bones, or muscle, but I did have a definite impression, and I remembered Alexander saying we should go with that impression. But it seemed too bizarre to be true.

"I have the feeling his eyes are crossed," I said, hesitating over a blurred image. "But it's not crossed eyes so much as disturbed vision."

"Elaborate if you can," said the moderator in a silky voice.

No clear picture came on my Screen, and then, suddenly, the words formed to describe what I wanted to say. "It's like looking at a mirror," I said. "Everything he sees is turned around."

The moderator's voice rang out triumphantly. "Exactly. He suffers from reversed vision."

There was a murmur of approval, but my own sense of achievement was clouded by the obvious coaching.

We had descended uneventfully to the area of the throat. The moderator's voice again became urgent. "What do you see there?"

I suspected something wrong with the boy's throat. It could have been a strep throat, tonsilitis, quinsy, any of a dozen things, but somehow I sensed a breathing difficulty. "Asthma, I think he's troubled with asthma."

After a whispered consultation, the instructor's voice rang out. "Correct again. You've scored one hundred percent."

The moderator had one more question. "This boy has a problem in school. Can you visualize it in your levels?"

I would have had to be the class idiot not to suspect. "He has a reading problem."

The moderator exultingly threw up his hands. "Eureka, you did it."

Grace Dade was the first to congratulate me. "You really hit it; the boy reads just the reverse of children with normal vision."

But one thing had impressed her more than the rest. "You got the asthma even though it wasn't written down."

"I may have picked it up from you."

She regarded me doubtfully. "I was not thinking about it or I would have put it down."

What had it all come out of, and why? Had I responded in some unknown way to a boy's subconscious appeal for help?

Not being a physician, I had so little knowledge of the boy's disability that I had to look up the medical term for it—dyslexia—and certainly had no way of helping him.

It was only a test. And having survived the test with no loss of ego, I was able to look around the room in a relaxed way and observe other students going through their paces. I was particularly interested in Lennie Weitz and the bumptious Joe.

Ralph Winters had passed with flying colors, correctly tuning into a woman with varicose veins. She was preparing for surgery, and he had somehow picked up that, too.

Linda Lockwood was sitting with her eyes closed, motioning with her hands as she visualized the case of a teen-age boy.

As I passed her, scouting about for Lennie, I overheard her say with a frown, "This boy has a blood problem. I see something wrong with the blood itself. I think it is leukemia."

Amazingly, she was correct.

In a distant corner, I found Lennie. There was quite a cluster around him and moderator Bob Smith. Isolated except for his girl friend, I saw Joe. His eyes were closed, and so was his mouth. He appeared in rapt meditation.

I craned my neck to follow Lennie's progress. He was sitting comfortably, legs spread out, a serene expression on his round face.

"He's already got about a dozen things right," said one astonished onlooker, "and he slept through it all. Can you imagine?"

The unidentified man of about sixty-five or so for whom Lennie was reading seemed virtually a basket case. He had a Pacemaker in his heart, diabetes, osteomyelitis (a deterioration of the bone), a plastic bubble for a stomach, one kidney, and one lung. And Lennie had gotten all this. It seemed incredible not only that he should have tuned in so precisely but that anybody could survive with so many things wrong with him.

And there was still more. Lennie was frowning over his subject's extremities.

"I don't see anything there," he said finally. "I think he's got a missing leg. It's like a wooden leg."

Again, he was right.

Lennie had accurately tuned into eighteen different ailments. It was hard to conceive of a human being wanting to go on with this much wrong with him. He would have to be of a melancholy disposition.

Bob Smith had not quite finished. "What else do you see about this man, about his personality or emotional makeup?"

The answer seemed obvious.

Lennie's eyes closed. He ruminated for a few moments, and I was afraid he had fallen asleep. But no, his lips were moving and framing words. He had put on the man's head, mentally.

"This man has a fantastic attitude. It's unbelievable. He's happy and bubbling, and enjoys every moment of his life."

Even Bob Smith seemed a little astonished. "That's very true," he said, "for this man is very close to me and I see him all the time."

How had the sleeping wonder done it?

His wife had wakened him when Alexander had repeated the cycles for getting into the levels, so Lennie had at least familiarized himself with the technique of reaching an altered awareness. The rest he had absorbed during sleep.

Beatrice, too, had gone through a surprising transformation. Her skin was a bright pink, and she appeared sunburned. There was no doubt in her mind how it had happened.

"In my passive scene from nature," she said, "I put myself on my favorite beach in Hawaii, and I felt the Hawaiian sun beating down on me."

I could hardly believe it, though it accounted for her healthful glow. "You mean, your thinking made you burn?"

"Not thinking, but actually feeling as if I was there. I could feel the burning heat of the sun, and its brightness. I didn't think it, I lived it."

Equally astounding were the white circles around her eyes, where she had visualized shielding sunglasses. It was truly a day of miracles.

I looked around the room now for the class iconoclast. Joe was still in the same chair, and a group had collected around him.

His moderator appeared to be smiling, and I was hopeful that Joe, at last, was behaving.

As I approached, Joe threw up his hands and looked around at the classmates who had clustered about him. His face wore an incredulous smile.

"I can hardly believe it. I came down to this guy's arm, and the moderator asks me to pick out what I see. And so I told him, I didn't see anything. 'I don't think he's got an arm,' and"—he motioned at the moderator—"and so he says, 'Right on, it was amputated.' "

He turned to me with a grin. "What do you think of that?"

After the last test case, everybody resumed their seats. Alexander seemed in good spirits. He even had a kindly glance for Lennie, awake now that the sessions were over.

Alexander's good humor seemed contagious. There were friendly smiles and embraces wherever one looked. My own mentor, Suzie, the shapely teen-ager, volunteered to help me with my cycles whenever I felt disposed. "Whenever you're tense, just visualize a nice relaxing massage and see how fast you loosen up."

Alexander delivered his peroration. "If it all ends with this class, whatever you gained in altered awareness may soon fade away, just as any physical exercises would become meaningless if you did not pursue them."

He paused for a moment, and his pale blue eyes benignly ran over the faces of the students. "I would suggest you practice going into your levels daily, and that you meet regularly to share your experiences. Most of you have discovered a latent ability. But if you don't use it—or if you abuse it—you soon lose it."

He was about to dismiss the class, when a lone voice called out from the rear of the room and a lone figure stood up. I groaned. It was Joe.

"Before this class breaks up," said Joe, "there is something I would like to say to every student here, and to every graduate, as well."

Joe seemed to stand straighter. His eyes shone. "You have all listened with great patience as I played the role of the skeptic, expressing doubts and criticisms, even as you were hopeful and optimistic."

His dark eyes traveled around the room, taking in each and every one of us. "I want to apologize for having been such a bloody bore, and for any discomfort I caused any of you." He paused. "Not until a few minutes ago, when I worked my test case and realized that I could actually tune into another person, did the light finally dawn. Please forgive me, all of you, and think of me as your friend, as I think of you."

As we moved to the exits, I remarked to Ralph Winters, "That was quite a thing Joe did."

Ralph nodded. "He had to release his ego, that's one of the hardest things for any of us to do."

We ran into a smiling Anne Francis on the way out.

"Somebody just told me," she said, "that the drapes actually were yellow."

I saw Alexander at the door.

"Well, what did you think of it?" he asked.

"I'm still trying to sort it out."

"Do you recall the poet John Donne's words, 'No man is an island, entire of itself. . . .' "

" 'Every man is a piece of the continent,' " I finished.

"And so," said Alexander, "as we dig below the surface, we find ourselves all part of the same consciousness."

Chapter 8

The Graduates

Even as a student, Linda Lockwood used her levels to program herself to success. On the third day of class, she slid into the room a few minutes after the lunch break and unobtrusively took her seat. She seemed flushed and breathing hard, as if she had been running. Her eye caught mine, and she nodded as if to tell me something.

Two hours later, over coffee, she cried, "It works, it works!"

Her rosy face radiated excitement. "I did it, I did it." She was practically jumping up and down.

"Did what?" I asked.

"I got the job. I just bowled them over."

"They didn't know it," she said exultingly, "but I had them all programmed, and it happened just as I visualized on the Screen of the Mind."

"Slow up," I said.

She drew a deep breath. "All right. I heard about this job yesterday, and didn't think I had a chance, but I made a call anyway, and they said to come in today before lunch. I wasn't sure I had the experience or qualifications. But I programmed myself anyway, going into my levels, and visualized the interview from beginning to end, even to putting the salary I wanted on my Screen. It was twice my last salary."

"And they agreed to it?"

"It didn't seem to faze them."

"So when do you start?"

"They said they'd let me know tomorrow."

She didn't have any doubt what the answer would be.

"I knew from my levels they would discuss it before coming to a decision. But I know what that decision will be."

"But how?"

"Because everything else happened just as I programmed it. They used the very phrases I had visualized."

"Such as?"

"Such as it was more than they had expected to pay, but this wouldn't rule out the right person."

"You might clinch the job if you moderate your demands," I said.

She gave me an almost pitying glance. "That's what impressed them—the salary I was demanding. They felt I must be good if I valued myself that highly."

She tapped my shoulder lightly. "And I owe it all to you. If not for this class, I would have never had the nerve to mention that kind of money."

The following day, I saw her slip out quietly. She returned by the afternoon session and promptly took her seat. Again she nodded, but this time with an emphasis there was no mistaking.

"Didn't I tell you?" she crowed later.

"Congratulations," I said, feeling that the enthusiasm generated by her programming might have contributed to her success.

As Alexander had pointed out, meditation had to be maintained regularly to be an effective tool. The divorced Linda, mother of two small children, had programmed herself to be married. She had even picked the date, May 23, only a few weeks off. At the weekly meetings of graduates, she spoke of her programming frankly, without appearing to notice the raised eyebrows or the half-smiles behind cupped hands.

A supremely confidant and noticeably slimmer Linda would not back down an inch. "Alexander said that when we programmed something we wanted, it might not always turn out as expected, but would still lead to something significant."

She had already seen it working. "I never truly liked my body. So I subconsciously reprogrammed my muscle tone and weight in my levels, saying that whatever I ate would only make me slimmer. I noticed my clothes feeling looser, and found I was losing a pound a day. I had injured my back in an auto accident. It had bothered me for seven years, restricting my movement. I began doing my exercises in my levels, bending way back, mentally, and soon found I could bend backwards in actuality."

Having a chronic sinus problem, Linda had been scheduled for surgery, but decided it would be an affront to her newly beautified body. "In my levels, I programmed myself to feel a sneeze clearing out any impurities causing infection in the sinus cavities and to open up the blocked passageways."

She even performed mental surgery, with the help of an ear, nose, and throat specialist, who was not consulted, and one of three Workshop assistants. "Helen, my physical assistant, helped the doctor perform the operation on the Screen of the Mind."

There was an awkward silence at this announcement, then somebody lightly asked, "How much did the doctor charge?"

Linda joined in the laughter. "It was the cheapest operation I ever had."

I was intrigued that she had three assistants when nobody had been programmed by Alexander for more than two.

"I just felt I needed more help than most people." Alexander, whose clarity she admired, was her mental assistant; a psychic friend, Sunny Orr, was her spiritual adviser.

Knowing she had such redoubtable assistants gave her a new confidence. "In my Workshop, I just put my feet up on a desk and greet my helpers, saying, 'I am glad you are here. I know you will help me and that you know everything I need to know.'"

Did Alexander know that he was her helper?

Linda's eyes twinkled merrily. "I didn't want to depress him."

Alexander was the first into the Workshop, and then Helen, a robust young neighbor. "She is always smiling and happy, always eager to help, and very supportive of my efforts." Sunny emerged with a glow of love around her head. "She is the most spiritual of the three, and I feel the presence of no one else when I am talking to her. She wants me to develop, and will patiently help me, through her understanding and love, to reach my ultimate goals."

Not all graduates were as enthusiastic as Linda. Some graduates acknowledged they still had a difficult time believing that anything was about to happen in their levels.

"Perhaps you don't go down into your levels thoroughly enough," Linda volunteered. As she visualized the rainbow, she rested a few moments at Blue, the loving color, and concentrated on its softness. On the countdown from twenty-one, she paused at nineteen, sixteen, and thirteen, to briefly scan her own skin, muscles, bones, nerves, pausing again at intervals of three until she reached one. "I tell myself that I will be relaxed and at peace to accomplish what I have to when I get to my Workshop." In her passive scene from nature her hearing, sight, and smell appeared to increase immeasurably, and she felt she had left the Beta brainwave pattern. "I don't need a Biofeedback machine to tell me I am in Alpha or Theta. I am so sensitized that strong smells make me uncomfortable. I sit at a window box, outside my Workshop, and feel the fresh, cooling breeze and actually hear the rustle of my hair as it gently falls back. Below my window, a garden is massed with flowers and heavily fragrant. Sometimes the man I expect to marry is in the garden, and he says, 'Why don't you come down and join me?'

" 'Not right now,' I say, 'as I have some work to do first. But I will be down after a while.' "

She visualized herself into her Workshop at the count of twelve, completely rested and ready to receive direction. "I get up from the window, take nine steps across the room, toward my bed, and at ten, eleven, twelve, measure off the steps to the platform. Then I sit down comfortably and put my feet up."

On the Screen, on the calendar of her mind, she visualized the date of her approaching marriage—that same May 23.

I was afraid Linda had discovered a new and dangerous toy, and I could see from their expressions that many from the class shared my view.

"You've got to be careful that you don't program the impossible and then suffer a letdown," I cautioned.

"Nothing is impossible," she said.

I hesitated a moment. "Has this young man asked you to marry him?"

"No, but he will."

She drew out a small sheet of paper and showed me a diagram of a calendar, with May 23 blocked out in a left-hand corner. The numerals were circled as though by the sun.

Though May 23 was still some weeks off, my uneasiness grew. "Keep in touch," I said. "I'd like to know how it works out."

Inevitably the heralded date arrived, and there was no sign of Linda. After two or three weeks I called, missing her several times before finally reaching her at home.

"Jerry and I broke up," she said drearily.

I had no heart to say, "I told you so."

"Did anything happen on that day?"

"What day?"

"May 23, your programmed date."

She thought awhile. "Not really."

"Anything at all?"

She searched her memory. "Somebody I had met over the phone, in a business way, called that day, and I'm going to dinner with him. But it's nothing. He's only a voice."

"What is this chap's name?"

She was at a loss for a moment. "Sid, Sid Bass. He's an insurance consultant. I haven't met him yet. The dance is next week."

"Well, have a nice time."

"I'll try," she said, almost in tears.

I hung up hastily. Poor Linda, once so high and now so low. But at least, she would come down to earth, approach her mind-training technique with circumspection, and hopefully rid herself of her assistants.

We had another session, at my home, a few days later, and Linda was not there. Ralph Winters, who was preparing to become a mind-training teacher, took over the proceedings.

"You did very well with your test case," he said. "How about doing a reading for us now?"

I was acutely aware of some two dozen people watching me closely. "I was lucky, and have no confidence I can repeat at will."

"Haven't you been practicing in your levels?"

"Not really. I'd rather remain the observer."

"Well, try anyway." He glanced about the room. "Anybody have a case?"

Attractive, fresh-faced Sahra Nichols, the mother of two teen-agers, raised her hand.

"Give him the age and sex of the subject," said Ralph.

I turned to Sahra. "If I get off on a tangent, just tell me and I'll stop."

She spoke in a low voice. "Could you tell me about a fifty-five-year-old woman?"

I visualized the colors of the rainbow, and was intrigued with the colors. I started to count down, and visualized a descending flight of stone steps that would take me into my Workshop, picturing a film of dust on the oblong table, chairs, television set, walkie-talkie, and even the window sills. I tried to visualize the raised platform, and a white screen with a light about it. I tried to imagine a fifty-five-year-old woman, but I could not see her face, only the gray of her head and the outline of her body. She was in bed, in a hospital.

"She is ill," I said. "Is that right?"

I could hear Sahra's soft, "Yes."

I had no idea where my next impression came from. "She has a lump in one breast?"

"Yes."

"This woman," I said with new conviction, "is your mother, and I see her getting well at this time. She has had a remarkable spiritual experience recently, in the hospital, and it has changed her outlook on life."

I opened my eyes, and was back in the room on the ocean without having reversed the rainbow, counted back, or used any other technique.

"You might check with your mother if it is she," I said, "to see whether she had such an experience."

Sahra looked at me solemnly. "I visited my mother in

the hospital two days ago, and she told me of her experience."

I had no feeling of elation. It all seemed so unreal, and I really had not accomplished anything or helped anybody, including Sahra, her mother, or myself.

"You demonstrated that it works," said Ralph reassuringly.

In succeeding sessions, graduates continued to report new wonders. With practice, they were able to eliminate the elaborate countdowns and go quickly into their levels, merely snapping their fingers or using the finger-thumb technique. Nearly everybody used the Screen of the Mind. It seemed to impart a sense of reality.

Like so many others, Eve Bruce chose herself as her first project. "If you're not all right," she said, "how can you help anybody else?"

Eve was practically a walking infirmary. She had an infection of the gums, a back so bad she was wearing a lift on one shoe, and had given up her favorite sport, tennis. She slept poorly, felt constantly tired and debilitated, with the black depression of the chronically fatigued.

The changes didn't occur all at once, but she dutifully reported each new miracle as it occurred. With Linda Lockwood conspicuously among the missing, Eve had become the life of the Alpha party. She would discuss her experiences with anybody who seemed interested, beginning with her first test case. She had been asked to check out a fifty-year-old woman. "She was blind, and suffered from tuberculosis and a chronic cough. She had a broken leg, and arthritis in both legs besides."

In her own case, X-rays had showed a deep infection of the gums, and her dentist had recommended removing three teeth and putting in a bridge.

"I went into my Workshop and put the inside of my mouth on my Screen, blowing up the picture so that it covered the entire wide Screen. I saw dark spots, just as the X-rays had indicated, realized they were the sites of infection, and visually cleaned them out. I actually saw them disappearing."

Eve returned to her dentist. He looked at the new

X-rays and shook his head. "Miracles do happen," he concluded.

Eve's back had bothered her since high school, when she took a bad spill, skating. She had been told that her spine was crooked, and only disc surgery would relieve her. The lift in one shoe evened up her hips.

But now she went to her levels again and put herself on her Screen. "I visualized my spine as perfectly straight and myself bending and flexing without pain as I skated and played tennis. I repeated this several times a day, always seeing my back as perfect, without strain. One morning, I felt no pain as I eased myself out of bed, nor as I showered and dressed. I put on my shoes, and my heart sank. I was standing, tilted to one side. And then, with a thrill, I realized that my lower spine was no longer uneven. I removed the lift, and I was perfectly straight and comfortable, just as I had visualized myself on the Screen of the Mind."

I had listened to this particular story with interest.

"And your tennis?"

She smiled. "I'm swinging better than ever."

"It seems to me," I said, "that if visualization works, all you have to do is visualize yourself as perfect and all your ailments drop away like a rattlesnake shedding his skin."

"When you've been using the wrong vibrations all your life, you have to get back on the track gradually." She smiled. "If a person had all this power of mind, he would never have attached himself to these illnesses in the first place."

I was struck by the way she put it. "Attached to illness?"

"Oh, yes, every actress knows that. You get a little unhappy, you're not working regularly, your personal life stinks, and the next thing you know you've picked up something."

But this was all in the past. This Eve had programmed the serpent right out of the Garden of Eden. For most of her adult life, she had been plagued with sleeplessness. "Now I have to program myself to stay awake."

She had first tried Alexander's technique of erasing numbers from one hundred down, blocking each number out with an "X." But she found it impractical. "I'd get down to zero, then start again. It was a bore."

She had made the discovery that the relaxing suggestions she gave herself to get into levels would sometimes nudge her to the edge of slumber. So she decided to repeat this technique in coaxing sleep. She remembered Lennie Weitz drifting off to sleep, and it reinforced her confidence. It resulted in her giving up trying to sleep but inviting it instead. "After a while, I'd fall asleep before I even got to the Workshop."

Eve had the feeling she was creating a dimension of the mind that could project into areas she had never dared think of before.

So when her mother called distraught one day to say that her pet Pomeranian had disappeared from the waiting room while she was in with her attorney, Eve told her to hang on while she went into her levels. The attorney's office was in Los Angeles, near Western Avenue, a main thoroughfare, and the dog could easily have been picked up by a pedestrian or run over by a motorist.

"In my levels," said Eve, "I saw two intersecting signs, Western Avenue and Beverly Boulevard. They were as clear as if I were standing next to them. I told my mother to go immediately to that intersection and she would find her dog."

An hour later her mother had called back happily. "She had found Fur on the sidewalk at Western and Beverly Boulevard, just lying on the corner, panting and waiting."

This new ability to help herself gave Eve an overall feeling of confidence in managing her affairs. Whatever the problem, she had a technique for coping with it, a newly unveiled layer of her mind that would serve in any emergency. It had not come at once, but had to be nurtured. "As I kept using my levels, the certain knowledge would come that this facility was now an integral part of me. I had a new dimension, and who knew how far it would carry me toward understanding my purpose in this life?"

Even with Eve, we all missed Linda and her charming ebullience. I had called several times but couldn't reach her. The summer passed traveling, and I returned home after Labor Day to find a message marked "Urgent" from Linda Lockwood.

Apprehensively I dialed her number.

She answered in a clear, resonant voice. "Oh, I'm so glad you're back," she said.

"You sound fine," I replied in relief.

"I never felt better," she said. "I'm getting married."

"When?" I concealed my surprise.

"In two days."

"To Jerry?"

"Oh, no." She laughed as if there had never been a Jerry. "I'm marrying Sid."

I thought for a moment. "The voice on the phone."

"I wasn't particularly smitten at first," she was saying, "but Sid's interested in the children and my happiness. And it gradually dawned on me that he was the one."

It was hardly my idea of a slow courtship. "You've known him less than three months."

"Don't you remember Alexander saying that sometimes we got what we wanted, but in an unexpected way? Well, May twenty-third, which I had programmed for marriage, was the very date that Sid first called me."

I couldn't help the feeling she had made it happen.

"Of course, but Sid's face finally filled out the picture on my Screen. The features had never been clear before, no matter how I willed it. I never saw Jerry's face there, even when I didn't see how it could be anybody else."

Naturally, I congratulated her.

"It'll be a simple wedding, with no one but family," she said. "And the seven of us will start on the honeymoon right after the ceremony."

I thought I hadn't heard right. "The seven?"

"Why, yes, Sid's three children and my two. I saw it all in my levels; it should be quite an experience."

With Linda safely disposed of, I had an abiding curiosity about the most curious graduate of all, and one day Lennie Weitz casually dropped by. He looked the same—rotund, placid, smooth-faced. His $80,000-a-year job had vanished when the firm's founder died, and he had started his own business, Heavenly Cosmetics, with a home-to-home service featuring a demonstration crew of attractive girls.

He smiled. "I call them the Heavenly Angels."

Headquartered in the San Fernando Valley, he already had spread out over several states and countries.

"It hasn't been easy," he sighed.

"I thought all you would have to do is visualize success and it would happen."

"You still have to work."

He was graver than I remembered him. "I'm older and wiser."

"As a result of your Alpha experience?"

"That and life." He frowned. "Actually, we never knew whether we were in Alpha or not, only that we functioned with new awareness in our levels."

I laughed. "Since you were sleeping practically all the time, you must have been in Theta."

"Theta-shmeta, it's all the same head."

He sank deep into the chair and patted his comfortable stomach.

"At first," he said with a distant look, "it was like a new toy. I'd put other people's heads on and know what they were thinking. I had two superiors in the business, and I wanted to know what they really thought about me. So I went into my levels, visualized their heads on my Screen, and slipped them on my shoulders."

It hadn't been a reassuring experience.

"How could you know for sure?"

"I tuned into very specific situations, and subsequently found these things were actually going on."

"If they hadn't liked you, they wouldn't have paid you that well."

"I was producing, working seventeen or eighteen hours a day."

He seemed suddenly introspective. "Sometimes it's better not to know how other people look at you. After all, they could be wrong."

"And so you do use it?"

"Just to look into my own head and know where I'm at, not to program anybody else, not anymore."

"Do you actually think you can influence other people?"

"Do I think so? Hell, I know so. A friend of mine had a kid who was shy and didn't play with the other kids. He worried about him growing up with nobody liking him. He was an extrovert type himself, and didn't understand that a person could be introverted and be comfortable with it. At my friend's request, I projected into the kid's mind, visualizing his head on my shoulders, and I programmed him to be outgoing, expansive, athletic, liking the company of other people."

"And it happened?"

"Almost overnight. The father thought I was Merlin the Magician."

"And was the boy any happier?"

"I don't know; he was different." Like so many fat people, Lennie was never solemn for long. His round face suddenly brightened. "Anyway, the father felt better."

"Do you think a person can use this advanced level of the mind to exert a bad influence?"

He looked at me as if I were some rare specimen.

"Why do you think I stopped fooling around with it?"

"But don't we resist suggestions inconsistent with our character?"

"If you got a million people around, putting other people's heads on, how do you protect yourself?"

"Couldn't you program yourself to think only healthy, wholesome thoughts, and so remain impervious to suggestions of a negative nature?"

"I don't know about that. But I do know it's wrong to invade another person's privacy." He sighed. "You don't need much education to know this is a terrible intrusion."

Lennie brooded for a moment.

His wife, Bea, never far away, said, "Tell him about the poet."

"Oh, yeah, the poet." He frowned. "This man wrote the most beautiful poetry, so warm and beautiful that we all wanted to meet him. It gave you a good feeling just to read him."

After a meeting had been arranged, they decided Lennie should descend into his levels and put the poet's head on— not wanting to write like him—but to know what to anticipate.

"Suddenly I get all this swearing and cursing and complaining. I felt sure I had made a mistake. It couldn't be the man who had expressed all these beautiful thoughts."

Then they met the man whose poetry they loved.

Lennie gave a shrug of his shoulders. "And do you know, if possible, this man was even worse than I had imagined him?"

So what had he lost?

His face became glum. "I was disappointed twice instead of once."

Perhaps it could be helpful in judging the people he had business dealings with?

He shook his head. "It's taking unfair advantage."

He was still grateful for the overall experience. "It helped me with my own head, and that's where it all starts. Looking into my own head, I could change those things I saw that I didn't like." His eyes twinkled. "I only hope I'm a better person for it—and sell more cosmetics."

After my first rush of enthusiasm, I did little, consciously, with my mind-training. Like most people, caught up in their daily affairs, I let things take care of themselves. However, from time to time, I would meditate, and it seemed to help.

Occasionally, for the fun of it, I would test the effectiveness of visualization, usually in a trivial way. One day, I was working out with twelve-pound dumbbells, when a strapping young athlete, a perfect specimen at six-two and 190 pounds, began prodding me good-naturedly.

"What," Scott Hubbell asked, "are you doing with those toothpicks?"

"They're heavy enough for me," I said, remembering he was a champion swimmer.

"I guess you're getting old."

"Not that old," I rejoined.

He gave me the cocky glance adolescents reserve for their decrepit elders.

"I'll bet I can hold up those toothpicks twice as long as you can."

I looked at this youthful Adonis, with his broad, deep chest, heavy shoulders, and powerfully muscled arms, and was about to turn away when I caught the gleam in his eyes.

My old competitive spirit suddenly flared up.

"You can't even hold them as long," I said brashly.

He made a jeering noise. "That's a horse laugh."

"You go first," I said, giving myself the advantage at least of knowing what I had to aim for.

He agreed readily, with a nonchalant smile, and swaggered over to pick up the dumbbells.

"Gosh," he said, "they really are toothpicks, aren't they?"

We decided the rules quickly. We would hold the watch on each other, checking off thirty-second intervals.

"That is," he said, "if you get to thirty seconds."

He flexed his arms easily, and his bare feet gripped the deck of the house. He took a deep breath, and with the dumbbells held out his arms rigidly at shoulder length.

It seemed to me, looking at him, that he could hold them forever.

At sixty seconds, however, his mouth had tightened a little, and at a minute and a half, his extended arms seemed taut and strained. His natural color had deepened a shade.

At two minutes, he was breathing noticeably, and his biceps quivered the least bit. At two minutes and fifteen seconds, with a muffled gasp, his arms dropped.

"There," he said, "beat that."

I had no idea what I could do. But on the Screen of my Mind, I plainly visualized two and a half minutes. I saw it clearly—2:30.

As I reached for the dumbbells, I visualized them not as twelve-pound weights, but as water wings, the air-filled type with which I swam when I was six or seven.

I was barely aware of Scott holding the watch. "Now, remember," he said, "if your arms drop even a little bit, you're through."

I took a deep breath, looked out on my passive scene from nature, the rolling Pacific, and extended my arms, shoulder-level. I closed my eyes to better visualize the water wings. They were large and airy, weightless. They were holding me above water.

Dimly, in the background, I heard Scott's voice. "Thirty seconds—sixty seconds—ninety seconds." He seemed less cocky, a little concerned. But the water wings were a little heavier, too.

"Remember," he barked, "no relaxing of arms."

Mentally I replaced the water wings with feathers. I thought to myself, "They are as light as feathers," and I kept repeating this thought. I saw the feathers clearly; they were ostrich feathers, and they billowed in the breeze.

They had no trouble staying up. Hazily I heard two minutes, and even with the feathers, something I had not programmed was happening. My arms still felt light, but the muscles, even the bones, were aching. I gritted my teeth, but asked casually, "What time?"

He said with disgust, "Two minutes and twenty seconds."

I held on for another ten seconds as he grudgingly called off two minutes and thirty seconds.

I slowly put the weights down and glanced up at a crestfallen Scott.

"I could have held on," I said, "for another hour or so."

Chapter 9

Why Miracles?

Where did these apparent miracles come from? How could a John Burnham reach into the atmosphere and influence a Kathy Bleser—if he did? How did a Dorothy Nelson presumably help a lady with failing eyesight, and that ailment return when she gave no sign of altered awareness? How did some program themselves for jobs, tests, romances, weight control, headaches, and others report a new inner peace and contentment, a new technique for handling everyday problems?

"How?" I asked the solemn-faced figure sitting across from me.

My old classmate Ernie Dade eyed me placidly through his steel-rimmed glasses. "Do you notice any changes in me?"

His beard seemed a little grayer, his hair a little whiter, his expression a little graver. I looked a little closer. Four years before, Ernie had gone on to become an instructor, and now, while not agenting, taught a course called MIND. As I thought of all this, I realized that Ernie had not really aged in terms of looking appreciably older. He looked wiser, more tranquil, and at peace with himself and the world. He had matured.

"I had to go into Alpha to check you out," I said half in jest.

He nodded wisely. "I was so elated with the changes in myself that I wanted to convert everybody. But I learned that people have to be ready for mind-training, they have to recognize a need and want to do something about it."

"And so why does it work?"

"People get into a state of altered consciousness where they tune into the Universal Mind, which knows everything."

I was disappointed that he had fobbed it off on this catchall.

"My life changed during those four days at the Ambassador," he said. "I first noticed the difference when we started to create our Workshops. I had a nice walnut-paneled study in mind, with chairs I could lounge in, just like my den at home. But in my levels, it seemed as if an outside force was determining what my Workshop should be like, and yet I realized at the same time it was coming out of me so that I could perform in a more efficient way."

He wanted solid oaken beams, and he got a plain white ceiling; plain walls instead of paneling, white marble floors instead of cozy shag carpeting. "I'd begin to install a grandfather clock with chimes, and it would become a stainless steel clock. The tables turned out to be practical glass and steel, even though I would have liked them in richly carved wood. It looked like an office, and I had no choice but to work there. My subconscious had decided what was best for me."

His attitude toward people underwent a revolutionary change. He had a tendency to classify people by their apparent importance. On a scale of ten, actress Anne Francis was a nine and a half. As a writer, I was a nine, and so was casting director Ralph Winters. Like so many people, he had a label for everything and everyone. This all changed when he observed sixes and sevens doing as well or better in their test cases than nines and tens.

"I wasn't sure I could do my test case, but I didn't think the others could do it either. How could that guy who snored through four days come up with anything? He had irritated me particularly, as it bothered me that he should lie around like that, distracting people. He was not very high on my list."

And then, suddenly, he saw the least likely people doing their cases handily, and he realized that he had been mistakenly assessing people all his life. "I had a number on everybody, and they really didn't have one unless you put it there."

Ernie's own test case had been a revelation. "You were involved in a way," he said.

"Was I your case?"

"A man sitting near you gave me the case; it was a former sea captain. When I got down to my levels, he looked like you, and I rejected it, thinking I had made a mistake. So I examined the body from the neck down only."

He saw the man's legs as swollen and purplish. He was in bed since he couldn't walk. He mentally put on the man's head, deliberately not seeing any face, and felt his eyes filling with tears. He began sobbing in bitter waves of self-pity.

When he came to the feet, he seemed to have made his first mistake. "I saw a big hole where a toe should have been, and said, 'He has the big toe on his right foot missing.'"

The moderator consulted his slip of paper. "No, it's the left foot."

While Ernie was trying to revisualize the foot, he overheard the muffled acknowledgment, "I put the wrong toe down; he's right."

He had correctly seen his subject building ship models, and that friends called him Cap. He had done very well, all in all, but one thing bothered him. Why had he seen my face on his subject's body?

Opening his eyes, he turned to the student whose case he had worked. "What does your friend look like?"

The man ran his eyes over the class. "Why," he said, "he looks like Jess Stearn."

While all this was interesting, it didn't seem enough to change one's life. So he had seen, paradoxically, a missing toe. It was a startling departure from normal awareness, yet what did it establish—an unexplained flash of telepathy or clairvoyance at most?

"Don't you see?" said Ernie eagerly. "I hadn't picked it up from the piece of paper or the friend's mind. I had tuned into the captain, never having seen or heard of him before. I recognized even then that this man had a need, and had subconsciously put it out into the atmosphere, where it became a part of the Universal Mind."

"In other words"—I turned to my own experience—

"John Burnham was able to help Kathy Bleser because she had subconsciously expressed a need for another doctor."

Ernie nodded eagerly. "I have seen it work a hundred times."

"But what did I have to do with it?"

"You were the dial that turned him onto the right frequency."

Ernie had struck me as rather dull and unimaginative. Yet he had shown a creative flair I would not have credited him with before. In his classes, he had innovated such visual aids as the Path of Opportunity, where the student could meet anybody he wished; the Time-Track, where he played back movies of his life; the Universal Bank, open 365 days a year, twenty-four hours a day, where he could deposit anything he didn't want and take what he wanted; and the Love Light, which enabled him to radiate the healing glow of love. Even the name of his course showed an unexpected originality —MIND—Man's Inner Nature and Development.

Ernie's students often formed a power circle, concentrating on somebody who urgently needed help. The person could be present or absent, known or unknown. This energy apparently moved with the burst of light. If one person could produce energy, perhaps several together would have that much more.

"In this circle," said Ernie, "the left hand is held palm up, the right hand over it and down, and we fill the space between with energy and call it love. You can actually feel the electricity as we connect hands on this high energy level."

Swinging from a tree, a thirty-year-old Tarzan had crashed with a heavy limb on top of him. He suffered severe internal injuries. "He went to the doctor," Ernie said, "and was told it would take six weeks to recover. Some seventy-five of us connected our hands, creating a chain of energy, and the end man took hold of his legs. He shot out of the chair like a rocket, and was better in three days." With all that energy, the room temperature had increased ten degrees.

Ernie's Show-and-Tell alumni sessions drew many skeptics as well. "One visitor asked us to tune into a middle-aged woman. A student gave him a rundown, listing her various disabilities, and mentioned she had a hip problem."

The man scoffed. "That's one thing she doesn't have. You people are just playing games."

Two days later he called contritely. "I passed on the reference to a hip problem to my mother-in-law. And, to my amazement, she confirmed her hip had been troubling her."

She had placed her hand on her hip and told him with a smile, "Anyway, you won't have to hear about it. The pain disappeared last Tuesday night at eleven o'clock."

At that precise time, the student had put her in a white light and beamed a message of perfect harmony and health.

It was a very pleasant story, and it may well have happened in just that way. But how?

Ernie looked at me almost wistfully, as if he wished I would stop playing the devil's advocate and work with him toward understanding this new awareness.

"She was like a ship sending out an SOS, and we tuned in. The son-in-law was the contact helping us to dial in, even though he knew nothing of the problem."

"Have you ever thought," I said, "that there might be a healing frequency in the atmosphere?"

"It might work that way, but you still need a reason, somebody wanting something badly, and somebody having the power to transmit in transmittable Alpha and Theta."

"And it could very well be sent to themselves."

He gave me a slow smile. "Let me tell you about the girl who couldn't stop eating potato chips. Her name is Carol Lawson. She is a sweet little actress, with an elfish charm, and potato chips, dipped in sour cream, are about the last thing she should train on if she wants to keep slim, svelte, and working.

"Her uncontrollable urge didn't even have the dignity of a major vice. Potato chips—how dreadful! She would stay off them for days, and then, just as she was complimenting her will power, her car would turn in to her favorite delicatessen. She tried therapy, and the therapist came up with a reason.

"Every time Carol got a rave review, she would get emotionally unsettled and head for the store.

"Now that Carol knew what triggered her miserable habit, you would think that it would vanish. Right? Wrong."

So Carol tried Ernie's MIND classes. As an actress, she could dramatize any situation, however fanciful or fantastic, however horrible or degrading. "Carol visualized herself as fat and sloppy, weighing eight hundred pounds, with the potato chips jammed in her mouth and the sour cream trickling down her chin. That was her picture of herself in her Workshop as she didn't want to be. She next saw herself slim and beautiful, a forest sprite, dancing gaily through meadows and woods, occasionally, with great delicacy, dipping into a bag of potato chips and disdainfully tossing one into the air. 'Potato chips, bah,' she said, 'who needs them?'"

I looked questioningly at Ernie. "And that did it?"

"Yes, she became the person she visualized on the Screen of her Mind, who could take them or leave them."

"No more potato chips?"

"She might take one once in a while, to demonstrate her control."

Something had been bothering me, a loose end, and I finally realized what it was. "Why potato chips?"

Ernie shrugged. "What difference does that make?"

"We still don't understand her problem totally."

Ernie smiled in his beard. "Her problem was not realizing that she had the means to alter her state of awareness."

Carol Lawson was very obliging. Bad reviews had never bothered her, only the good ones, and this was enough to water down the sweet smell of success.

"Why did you react adversely to only good notices?" I asked.

"I couldn't handle the compliments. Deep down, I obviously didn't think I was as good as they said, and so I would punish myself."

Therapy and Alpha-training combined to eliminate the habit. "In therapy, I saw the problem intellectually, and in my levels, I got in touch with my feelings about myself as an actress and found myself saying, 'I deserve these notices or I wouldn't be getting them.' "

Basically it had been an emotional rather than an intellectual problem, and she had solved it emotionally, on the super-aware subconscious level.

There was still the unanswered question. Why potato chips? Why not candy, cake, pie, or ice cream?

Carol's laugh was like a bell. "I don't know."

I thought of all the brainwashing we unsuspecting mortals are subject to. "Do you remember that potato chip ad, with actor Bert Lahr saying you can't eat only one?"

"Oh, yes," said Carol, "I heard it often."

Ernie, like Carol, didn't think it mattered as long as she no longer stuffed herself with them.

I thought him rather smug. "You have nothing but successes, I imagine?"

Ernie smiled thinly. "Wrong. The same thing doesn't work for everybody. Each person has to shop around to find what works for him."

"And his assistants, can't he call on these powerful beings?"

He mused a moment, his chin in his hands. "In failure, often we learn more than with success. There are right and wrong suggestions. Some help the individual get at the problem, others keep him from unlocking his own inner awareness. One of my biggest failures was an overweight nurse named Mary Olson. She had a lovely face, but she weighed close to 180 pounds. Being a nurse, she had many diets available to her. They were good diets, and they worked with most people, but not with Mary Olson. She came to my class, having heard that many students had lost the poundage they wanted. She went into her levels and visualized the various methods other students had successfully used to lose weight. She put herself up on the Screen, in a black frame, exaggerating her own obesity so that she looked positively repulsive. She saw herself in the white frame, as she wanted to be. She visualized a date a month off and mentally inscribed on this calendar the weight she aspired to be on that date. She even put herself on a scale and saw the needle stop at 132 pounds. How could she miss?"

The days came and went, then weeks and months, and Mary hadn't lost an ounce. She considered for a moment that Ernie might be a charlatan, then dismissed the thought, knowing that he was not particularly concerned about money. Perhaps the course was inadequate, but then she remembered all the students for whom it had worked. She finally eliminated every negative but herself. She decided to go into her levels, put herself on the Screen, and run a motion picture of her life, Ernie's Time-Track. She saw herself as a small child, then a growing girl, a teen-ager, slim and lovely, first dating boys.

"When she discovered that young men didn't ask her out just to look at her, she was tremendously shocked. Unconsciously, she did what many attractive girls do when sex becomes offensive; she began programming herself to become unattractive. She started putting on weight. In the last scene of her movie, she saw herself as she now was, attractive enough, feature-wise, to attract men she wanted, but with the sort of body that would not stimulate overtures unless she desired them."

Mary's unconscious mind had done what it was programmed to do without letting on to her conscious mind what it was, and now, uncannily, it did something else. Unpredictably, as she opened her mind to the infinite, there appeared on her Screen of the Mind the face of a doctor who had addressed her graduating class in nursing and invited the young nurses to come to him for help if they ever needed it. That had been a long time ago, and it may have been a routine remark, but Mary Olson was not about to pass up this revelation.

She had gone to many doctors and tried many diets. She had been on amphetamines, to kill her appetite and boost her energy, and on diuretics, to eliminate fluids. And she still hadn't lost a pound. But never before had a doctor showed up on her Screen. It had to mean something.

The doctor didn't remember her, but he smiled encouragingly. "And what is your problem?"

"I have terminal obesity," she said. "Either it will kill me or I'll kill me." She looked at him imploringly. "You said you would help me."

He prescribed a weight-reducing pill with no amphetamines in it and said that as a nurse she knew enough to handle her own calorie intake. Mary decided she needed reinforcement, and returned to Ernie's class. She visualized herself in the Universal Bank.

"I went into my cycles, and saw myself depositing forty pounds, payable in three months."

The imaginary teller objected. "How about depositing a little at a time? You know how you are."

"No, I want a receipt for the entire forty pounds."

Reluctantly he handed her the receipt. "As you will."

Mary continued to program herself, even as she took the diet pills. "I visualized myself on a crash diet, and I fasted for the next twenty-eight days." In that time, incredibly, she ate only one hamburger, two eggs, and six boiled shrimps. She drank coffee, some fruit juices, and took vitamins. "I visualized myself rested and alert and I was never tired, and I had an intensive care patient for twenty days of this time."

With all this, she only lost seventeen pounds.

She kept visualizing the weight she wanted to be on the programmed date. She went back to eating, but only wholesome foods, cutting out the "junk" food—candy, potato chips, soft drinks—telling herself she would not allow her body anything fattening while she felt fat. She lost steadily, and on the programmed date she was the programmed weight.

She was now a shapely 137 pounds, and found her poundage no longer a problem as long as she kept reinforcing her slimness in her levels. "All you have to do from time to time is reaffirm the deep relaxation that allowed your body and mind to solve the problem. Looking at things realistically, you learn to enjoy people for what they are and for what they contribute. It is pleasant to be involved romantically on this basis, without putting up a lot of barriers."

Her own faith was renewed by the revolutionary mind work she saw being done in hospitals. "Some of the younger doctors, and a few older ones, are now advising bedridden patients to take a few minutes off three times a day from television, or brooding about themselves, to meditate and think of themselves as being well.

I was delighted to hear one doctor tell a patient, 'Think of the tumor and see it going away.' "

When a patient said plaintively of his ailment, "It's killing me," a mind-oriented doctor would wince. "Don't tell me that," he would say. "Tell me only where it hurts, and tell yourself you're getting well."

It was heartening to encounter young people like Carol Lawson and Mary Olson, who had done something about problems that disturbed the even course of their lives and blocked their potential as happy, healthy human beings. Still the cases were not the same, and there was a distinction I found puzzling.

"Carol Lawson knew what caused her to overeat," I pointed out, "and yet it didn't help her."

Ernie leaned forward and his eyes gleamed. "Carol knew on a conscious Beta level, Mary's realization came in the Workshop, where the subconscious mind could very readily attack a subconscious problem. Once there was a recognition of what was wrong on this level, the weight was lost. And, subsequently, this also happened with Carol. Only the timing was different."

Anybody who could harness his mind could meditate, and almost anybody could get into Alpha with the proper meditation. It was not some occult abstraction belonging only to the Yogis of the mystic East. It was a definite function of the ordinary mind. All that was required was the wish, and a technique to implement this wish.

People were often in Alpha or Theta without realizing it, particularly creative people who deliberately sought to contact mind, body, and spirit. Shakespeare, Shelley, and Keats all visualized as they created, as did the great inventors, Thomas Edison, Faraday, Watts. But not everybody was a genius, with a natural well of inspiration, and it took a calculated effort for lesser mortals to attain corresponding heights.

Alpha-training added a new dimension to meditation. In Yogic meditation, one began with a seed thought to still the restless mind, then allowed the mind to idly drift. The original image might have been a sad-eyed Christ, a Lincoln or Gandhi, Leonardo, Moses. And this image seldom changed in ordinary meditation. But in Alpha visualization, drawing on both memory and imagination, the expanded creative faculties often had a Lincoln or a Gandhi moving through life.

Even as I meditated, I wondered if these were actual scenes dredged out of the Universal Mind or sheer fantasy? In any case, it was very real to me, adding a new and broader dimension to my imagination. Instead of drawing on memory alone, I now visualized historic characters and watched them grow before my eyes. Even a fearsome Jehovah smiled occasionally, moderating his wrath at a stiff-necked people.

Different people, of course, were affected differently, depending on where they were in life and where they wanted to get.

In Alpha meditation, Indian Chief George Pierre, a former Congressman, experienced a marshaling of the mind in one disciplined effort. After six days with instructor Mark Beshara's Mind Probe One in Beverly Hills, the wounded forty-eight-year-old veteran of World War II was able to raise his right arm over his head and clench three fingers of that hand for the first time in thirty years. "What the course enabled me to do was to release that segment of the mind that had negative control over the muscles of my arm. Most people go through life without using their minds in totality, and I was one of them."

His visualization had relieved a spastic condition, without curing it, and given his arm increased movement, without giving it full mobility. "Because of the motor damage I sustained from a gunshot wound in the head, I improved to the fullest potential the mind alone could manage."

Some thought that George Pierre might have progressed even further by not limiting his own mind power.

Beshara, a doctor of philosophy, pointed out: "On the first night of training, George Pierre opened and closed his right hand under its own power. On the fourth night, he reported the gradual return of sensation in the right hand and arm. On the sixth day, he used his right hand and arm while driving for the first time in thirty years. That very afternoon, before the entire class, he lifted his right arm (classified as permanently handicapped) over his head. And within three days after completing the training, he reported that he had lifted a fifty-pound weight three times with his right arm."

Alpha teachers were often students caught up in Messianic waves of helping mankind. Fortunately, many of these teachers subordinated the fee structure to their own spirituality. Pat Patrick, teaching at Brentwood Youth House, Los Angeles, called her course Finding and Using the Higher Self, and her tuition fees were so slight they hardly paid the bills. "I like to think that the people I help will pass it on."

Her classes stressed her own discoveries. "Fundamentally, success in life is a matter of finding an open door and knowing yourself well enough to take advantage of the opportunities on the other side of that door."

"You learn with Pat," said Byron Meyers, a Hollywood screen director, "to stop dwelling on the negative. In digging up past mistakes and reverses, you keep them alive."

Originally, the youthful Meyers had experimented with his new powers as a sort of ego trip. "I'd practice concentrating on getting parking spots in busy streets, casing out somebody with an ulcer at thirty paces, and generally demonstrating how super I was. Meanwhile, I wasn't doing anything about the major problems in my life."

I had known the young director for some time, well enough to know of his quest to relate the business of making a living with a need to feel he was a part of some broader purpose. When I first met him, he had a hip problem and walked with canes. He was jobless, single, alone, and unsure of himself. He had now thrown away the canes, was married to a most attractive girl, and was doing what he wanted—making pictures with a theme.

Beyond all this, he had gained one thing which had put him on an easy footing with the world. He had become calm. "Before this calmness came over me, I was upset all the time, discouraged, unemployed, and broke. Now I'm doing what I like most and making money at it. And I've grown to realize there's nothing wrong with material rewards as long as they're a by-product of what you're doing, not the whole thing."

He had become an advocate of Alpha expectancy. "It

isn't enough to want something and say you want something. You have to have faith that it will happen."

Faith was not an abstraction. It produced a mind state supplanting Beta thinking with the creative energies of Alpha-Theta.

"You have to climb out of a narrow intellectual trap built on fear and false starts. You need a clear channel, not only to what you are and what you want to be, but to connect with other people and the physical world itself."

He had become something of an amateur healer, his hands transmitting heat energy across a room. "I wouldn't call myself a real healer, but I have had some success." He had wanted his mother to knit something for him, but her hands were too crabbed with arthritis to ply the needles. "I put my hands on hers for five minutes, and her knuckles loosened up. A week later she finished my sweater."

He looked like anything but an esoteric figure.

"There's nothing supernatural about any of this," he said, "it's the most natural thing in the world. I've seen these Eastern Indian Yogis and their hippie cultists try to transform life into some sort of deistic nonsense, with their beards, diets, sacred trappings, and exercises, all wearing the same uniform of separateness as they pride themselves on being different by working free fourteen hours a day for some guru, and sleeping on a pad in a dirty room, and paying for the privilege. They babble about being spiritual and unmaterialistic, but are only dirty and unkempt, afraid to face up to any challenge. They don't know what faith is, and their calm is the calm of the grave. They may as well be dead, for they're not alive. They talk about the Breath of Fire, the heavy-breathing exercise that's going to give them this exalted Kundalini that makes them at one with the oneness, and then they live like robots. It's all hot air."

They had visited him in droves, these youthful remnants of the hippie decade, hoping to bask in the light of a junior guru.

"One of the young girls," he recalled, "had broken her foot and was put in a cast. I put my hand on her cast and threw light around her. In two weeks, the foot had healed and she was able to remove the cast."

They vanished like the fog before the wind. "They didn't want anything real in their lives. When they were confronted with a force that could actually accomplish something, it blew their minds. They would rather play word games with their guru."

In the middle years, landscaper Ralph Laird of Downey, California, had also attained this inner tranquillity that Byron Meyers spoke of so calmly. All his life he had been afflicted with severe migraine headaches, and now there had been only one in four years. "It's a matter of controlling yourself at a deeper, unconscious level," he had decided. Laird seemed so calm that it was difficult seeing him as the once irascible figure he had painted himself.

He laughed easily. "At one time, every little thing bothered me. But as you meditate in your levels, visualizing the ordinary problems of the day on your Screen, you insensibly begin to feel at one with the universe and draw on this unlimited source."

He looked up with a smile. "How can some cranky customer rattle the universe?"

He seemed so calm that I wondered what cataclysm had caused his only migraine attack.

"I simply reverted. Somebody insisted I do a week's work in two days, and I blew up." He smiled ruefully. "I paid for it dearly, and I swore never again. Without self-control, we have no way of controlling anything."

With Ernie Dade, it was knowing yourself; with Byron Meyers, inward calmness; Ralph Laird, self-control; and with twenty-seven-year-old Michael Ellard, a Vietnam veteran, having a technique he could call on when needed.

Michael felt himself directed to Pat Patrick's class. He was on a boat, fishing, when he fell and revived an old rib injury. He cried out in pain, and a stranger, claiming some knowledge of psychic healing, passed his hands over him. "Stay quiet and believe you will be well." Very shortly, the pain passed. Michael thought of it as a miracle. The stranger said it was as natural as rain.

Michael had the Vietnam blues. He had seen comrades blown up, his best friend die mangled in his arms.

Horrible nightmares woke him up in a cold sweat. The best job he could get was driving a delivery wagon. Then somebody told him of Pat Patrick's class. "My experience on the boat had made me receptive. I went once and was hooked." He was inspired by graduates who had programmed themselves out of headaches, depression, tension, and whatever it was that was ailing them. He felt himself coming together in his levels, becoming a part of the universe, and that brought him back, ironically, to the community.

He had become a changed person, a success, with the love of life in his eye. He had shed his hippie uniform and was immaculately dressed, with a handlebar mustache and an easy way of talking.

His first test of his new awareness came while studying for a FCC license to repair television station equipment. There were four exams. "I got perfect hundreds in two, and ninety-six, ninety-seven in the others. I would go into my levels, visualize mathematical formulas on my Screen of the Mind, and commit them to memory. I programmed myself to remember by merely putting my first finger and thumb together, just as I did while driving, to keep fresh and alert."

He had visualized the job he now held, with United Press International, and the job interview as well.

Suddenly nervous about the interview with UPI's chief engineer in San Francisco, he telephoned his instructor, asking her to be with him in spirit.

Pat promised to go into her levels for the interview and surround him with a little white light on her Screen of the Mind.

"Just visualize the interview before you fly up from L.A.," she told him, "and see it successfully concluded."

The chief engineer was waiting at the airport.

"I picked him out immediately. He was in his early thirties, with red hair, and freckled, just as I had seen him in my levels. I went up to him immediately and shook his hand. I could see him wondering how I had recognized him without a description, but he didn't say anything."

The interview went swimmingly. Michael felt completely in possession of himself, yet that he was being controlled to do the right thing. "Before the man asked a question, I could anticipate what it would be, and so have my answer ready."

The engineer came to his key question. "What is your reaction to being called out at all hours?"

Michael had expected the question. "I would consider it part of the job."

The engineer gave him a satisfied smile. "You've got the job."

He called Pat in some elation when he got back to Los Angeles. "I felt you were really there."

She paused a moment, then said in a puzzled voice, "What was blue? I kept seeing blue during the interview."

He laughed. "My new boss was wearing a blue suit, blue shirt, blue tie, and blue socks. The room had blue walls, and on the wall was a picture with a blue background."

Nobody knew how Michael did it. In one week alone, he piled up fifty-six hours' overtime, and in a four-day stretch had only five hours' sleep. "They called me the Martyr at the office. But all I would do is go into my levels, putting my finger and thumb together, and tell myself I just had eight hours' sleep."

He had so much energy that, besides his servicing duties, he branched off into photography and dark room printing. He was also known as the Eager Beaver.

He looked as if he didn't have a care in the world. "I even visualized myself out of my nightmares, and the whole nightmare of the war went with it. I just told myself in my levels that the war was over for me—and my dream center got the message."

How many hours had he spent with psychiatrists?

"None. Pat suggested I release the nightmares, and I never had another one."

"Just like that?"

He made a circle of his thumb and index finger. "Just like that."

It was a most remarkable recovery. Had the subconscious suggestion been a dagger knifing sharply into the unconscious mind responsible for the memory pattern sustaining the nightmares? It seemed that way.

At twenty-seven, Michael was understandably full of himself and his new ability. He pointed to his attractive brunette wife, who had also taken the course. "Margaret had a bad back from a railroad crossing accident in which somebody was killed, and I have worked on that, helping get rid of the pain."

Margaret nodded her agreement. "Michael would take himself into his levels at the same time I did, and we would both visualize my back as being free of pain. It really has helped."

I couldn't resist. "How did you know which of you really did it?"

They laughed. "We are in each other's mind all the time, so it's all one."

He had even become something of a psychic detective. Somebody had called to say that a dear friend had disappeared while surfing and they feared for his life.

"They asked if I could help find him," Michael said, "and I went into my levels. At that instant, I saw him floating in a bed of kelp two hundred feet from the shoreline, and I named the cove, just off the Pacific Coast Highway."

And there they found his friend, drowned while surfing.

Had Michael Ellard had any idea why this meditation worked for him when nothing else seemed to—not friends, family, church, or school? Was it the mere technique, or was it this feeling previously mentioned of being controlled by a power outside himself?

His eyes kindled, and he replied so quickly that I wondered if he was in his levels.

"The subconscious mind is the controlling factor. In this mental sphere you visualize and create what you want, and every cell of your body responds to this unspoken effort."

Chapter 10

Star Pupils

"Call Carolyn Carroll," said Ernie Dade. "She not only got rid of sugar diabetes by going into her levels, but she's got medical records to prove it."

That seemed a tall order. I could understand relieving headaches and tension, even peptic ulcers, through the relaxing medium of Alpha-like meditation. But how did one radically change a condition of the blood, the blood sugar itself?

"Carolyn has all the information," said Ernie, "including the name of the doctor."

Carolyn Carroll was slim, youthful, attractive, with reddish-brown hair and a quick laugh. She lived in Encino, in the San Fernando Valley, the bedroom of Los Angeles, with her husband and two small children. She had been a professional dancer and still moved with a certain lithe grace.

"Oh, yes," she trilled in a musical voice, "I not only visualized myself out of diabetes, but out of two lumps in my breast that the doctor had been concerned about."

"Who is your doctor?" I asked.

"Doctor Charles Farinella; he's been the family physician for years."

"What kind of doctor is he?"

"A general practitioner, an M.D.," she said with the suggestion of a smile. "He's the administrative head of Golden State Memorial Hospital."

"Was he sure that you had diabetes, and not something that simulated it?"

"He took a blood sugar count, and it was two hundred and forty-seven—considerably above what it should have been—and he told me I had diabetes. It was quite a blow since I had gone in for my annual checkup not thinking I had anything wrong but a small cyst in my breast. This was removed and turned out to be benign."

She wasn't put on insulin immediately. "The doctor, a nutritionist, decided to improve my diet, cut out the starches, and see if I would respond."

She made no substantial improvement. Then she and her husband, Eddy, began Ernie's mind course in February of 1973. Two small cysts had reappeared and added to her concern.

Eddy, an actor-writer, had a dust allergy and needed corrective shots regularly. "Can you imagine an actor with a runny nose?" Carolyn laughed.

On the sixth and last day of the course, she became her own test case. "As long as I was putting anybody on the Screen of the Mind, I thought I'd try to help myself, on the theory that charity begins at home."

Carolyn went through her cycles, scanned her muscles, nerves, circulatory system, seeing herself as she never had before. She noted the two lumps in her breast and visualized the sugar floating around in her bloodstream. Then she visualized herself as she wanted to be—perfect. And then, in her Workshop, she proceeded, mentally, to heal herself. She showed remarkable resourcefulness. She didn't rely exclusively on herself or her assistants; she summoned the man she trusted, above all—her attending physician, Dr. Farinella.

"Now, Doctor," she visualized, "I want you to treat me in such a way that the sugar diabetes will disappear and the cysts will be gone. Do whatever you can to make me perfect." And then as an afterthought, "And while you're at it, Doctor, please lower my cholesterol count since, as you know, it's a little higher than it should be."

The doctor examined her, in her levels, and passed a hand over her, and said she was now in perfect condition, with her whole body in order, and that she should be re-examined in ten days.

All this, of course, was news to Dr. Charles Farinella. However, he was very happy to see his pretty patient when she came in for her appointment.

He checked for the lumps, and they were gone. The

cholesterol count was safely down, and the sugar count was below the diabetic level of 170, but barely. She was not quite satisfied, and decided to keep programming the sugar count down.

I wondered how much she had told the doctor.

"Everything," she said gleefully. "He is a very open man and feels, like many doctors, that the mind can get people sick and the mind can get them well."

"Did you tell him about his role?"

She laughed. "I wouldn't keep it from him."

He had chuckled tolerantly. "Someday people will walk into a drugstore, slip a coin in a machine, and get their individual aura."

Eddy, too, had profited. He had examined his nose carefully, visually removed it, and peered into it. He started talking to it, soothing the enlarged nasal passages. He saw himself throwing away the needle, no longer needing the shots to control his problem.

I still had to ask, "And what happened to his nose?"

"It cleared almost immediately, and he's never taken another shot."

Carolyn's family began relying on her for miracles. Her father, a safety engineer, had mislaid an important report and had vainly searched his office.

"I went into my levels," Carolyn said, "and saw the report in a file cabinet, back in a drawer, in a dark place."

Her father couldn't think of anything answering this description. But as a last resort, he looked into a dark place, an office closet, pulled open a drawer, poked in the back, and there found the missing report.

Carolyn's mother had a mole on her upper chest and asked if Carolyn could do anything about it.

"Sure, Mom," said Carolyn.

She was in her levels two or three times a day anyway, programming her blood sugar down, so it wasn't much to work on her mother as well.

"Every day, I'd mentally peel off a little of the mole."

One day soon, her mother called excitedly. "Carolyn," she cried, "My mole just flaked off."

The next day, her sister phoned and asked, "How are you with warts?"

The Carrolls even programmed the house they wanted to buy. "Eddy and I went into our levels, and saw a yellow and white house, with pine paneling, a step-down living room, a step-up dining room, and open-beam ceilings."

For nine months, they visualized the house, and finally the very house they saw turned up. There was only one discrepancy. Everything else was as they had visualized it, but instead of being yellow and white on the outside, the house was a dirty green. They couldn't stand it. On moving in, they immediately repainted it yellow and white.

A neighbor came by and admired their taste.

"Do you know," he said, "that's the exact color it was before the last people painted it green six months ago?"

They told Ernie Dade about this experience.

"You see," he said, "you should always scratch beneath the surface!"

Carolyn was understandably elated. With constant programming, her sugar count had dipped to 134, a safe mark, and life had opened up new horizons as vast as infinity. She saw the tremendous implications in programming youth. "They should start teaching kids this new awareness in junior high and high school. They would begin to know who they were and what they want of life. It would be a lot healthier than tripping on drugs."

Dr. Farinella, as I had surmised, was considerably more cautious than his patient.

Yes, she had had diabetes. No, she didn't have it anymore. But it was no miracle, it was completely predictable, knowing the patient and the impact of proper nutrition.

"Carolyn is inclined to be enthusiastic," said her doctor, "but I have to be scientific and objective. We changed her diet, took her off carbohydrates, got her to lose weight, and with this control she got better."

I had never heard of diabetics recovering so rapidly and completely.

"Didn't mind control have anything to do with her getting well?"

"Of course," he said, "she psyched herself out. But there's nothing unusual about that. We all know that attitude is a decisive factor in success in any field, including patient recovery. The champion in sports, the golfer or fighter carries in his mind the picture of his winning, not permitting the specter of defeat to cloud his thinking."

"You mean, the great golfer visualizes the perfect swing before making his stroke?"

"It happens all the time; there's nothing new about it. Doctors know that the will to get well is of extreme importance."

I thought of the deep, relaxed state almost symptomatic of Alpha-thinking. "Don't people heal better when they're relaxed?"

"Naturally, for tension is frequently a barrier to the body's own healing process. If a person's in a state of deeper relaxation, the autonomic defense mechanisms naturally act more efficiently."

"Well, couldn't this have occurred in Carolyn Carroll's case?"

There was a momentary hesitation.

"We live in a very turbulent world," he finally said, "where the emotions are constantly being challenged. Obviously, if a person becomes more stable internally, his autonomic functions will respond to a greater degree. Science is pretty well convinced today that the human system is like an electromagnetic field. But, as a physician, I have to look at these things very skeptically, while not denying they may happen."

"And you are sure that Carolyn is no longer diabetic?"

"As long as she watches herself, there is no reason for her to take insulin."

Carolyn was understandably puzzled by the doctor's professional reserve. "But I am eating whatever I want now, including carbohydrates, and my blood sugar is normal." She thought a moment. "And how did the lumps in my breast disappear?"

Not being a doctor, I didn't have the answer.

Students eagerly discussed their new awareness, their new ability to relate to people, to be gentle on themselves, more productive and creative, earning more money and enjoying it more. Gone were the fears and heartaches of yesteryear, bringing an optimism that made life not only tolerable but exhilarating. I kept hearing: "I had a new attitude."

"I saw that I was what was wrong with my marriage."

"I was able to get the job I wanted and keep it."

"I had confidence in myself for the first time."

"I was able to love and be loved."

These responses were subjective, indwelling, and could hardly be considered except in terms of the students' own feelings. You either accepted them or you didn't. There was no way of putting a definitive finger on these emotional changes. And I supposed that was why test cases usually concerned specific body condition, already identified, and why the most substantial support of Alpha-Theta changes was found in the relief of physical illness.

In the very nature of a reported recovery, there were the ingredients of hope, despair, near-tragedy, and then a triumph of faith that carried the testimonial of a sound body and mind.

Arlene Scott was no chronic complainer, no hopeless neurotic, but a healthy housewife and mother of thirty years. She had raised three daughters while helping her husband run the family business. "I really enjoyed operating a motel, but I did occasionally resent that I could not have some part of my life just for myself. There were many things I wanted to do, and I yearned at times for some privacy, for peace and solitude."

Who is to say how these coupled resentments and yearnings expressed themselves deep in Arlene Scott's subconscious mind? But in any case, in March of 1973, at age fifty-three, her body told her something was wrong. "I began to experience almost constant headaches." She thought it might be changing vision, the menopause, thyroid imbalance. But medical examination ruled out these possibilities, and the headaches became worse. Severe pains developed in the shoulder blades, the left arm, and the left side of the neck and face. She thought rest might help, but the pain made sleep virtually impossible.

In December of 1973, the Scotts took over a motel in the Milwaukee area. But Arlene Scott found, with sinking spirits, that she could no longer help her husband. "I had hoped to do the bookkeeping, but was unable to even bend my neck."

She was also unable to perform the household chores. In her despair, she addressed herself to prayer: "Not as I will, Oh Lord, but as you will, thy will be done for me and my affairs."

She continued to deteriorate. She felt a prickly sensation in the upper shoulders and neck, and could sleep only by adjusting her neck at a certain angle on a rubber cushion. A neurologist put her in the hospital for extensive tests. There were X-rays, brain scans, spinal taps, cervical bed traction, a headache diet, tranquilizers. "They showed some arthritis and a tendency toward diabetes." But nobody knew for sure what was wrong.

She was given prescriptions for four types of medication. These didn't help, and she begged the neurologist for anything that would give her relief. He told her she would have to reenter the hospital. As she was resisting this idea, she happened to catch Meditation Institute's Bill Schwartz on Milwaukee television, reciting the wonders of meditation and inviting the public to an open workshop. Since she hadn't driven for months, her husband took her to the seminar.

She soaked up Schwartz's words like a sponge. "For the first time in my life, I learned how to completely relax and build a positive attitude." She rejoiced in her meditation. "I felt the rush of the white surging waves of emotions through my body and felt completely in tune with the Infinite Intelligence. I felt nourished by the spirit within, and heard clearly the voice of intuition."

After one session, relaxing at will without medication, she was able to control her headaches. Instead of entering the hospital she entered Schwartz's thirty-hour course. For Arlene Scott, grounded in Christianity, it was a spiritual revelation. "I experienced the light of Christ flooding through my consciousness, dissolving all acid thoughts, recognizing that thoughts of resentment and ill-will tear down the cells of the body and poison the blood. I felt as though Jesus Christ was saying to me, 'Be thou healed; thy sins are forgiven.' I felt the presence of an invisible power that protected me and all those I love, and brought me every righteous desire of the heart."

Her release of tension, blocking the free flow of mind energy, had opened a door to her deeper self. "God's love poured through me in an irresistible current, letting go of worn-out conditions and worn-out things. Divine order was established in my mind and body. I was given the power to change any unhappy conditions. In the place of sorrow, appeared joy; instead of sickness, health; instead of lack, plenty."

God, the Infinite Intelligence, the Universal Mind, the Master who was the Messenger, all these were the inexhaustible reservoirs into which she hopefully tapped. But as ethereal as it appeared, there was still a technique, still a way of getting to her inner being and communicating. "I found that happiness must be earned through perfect control of the emotional nature. In meditation, I take my problems like ships over a calm sea. Every cell in my body feels regenerated, and I give thanks for the feeling of radiant health and endless happiness."

But this had to be constantly nourished. After her course, Arlene Scott came down with a two-day headache, alarming her all the more since she felt she had vanquished this problem. And then she realized that she had not meditated for days. "I went into meditation, completely relaxing, and within thirty minutes my headache was gone."

With Arlene Scott, tuning in had led to a religious experience latent in her past. Some had a spiritual release without being religious, and still others felt almost a physical communion with the world.

"My love affair with the world," said Betty Perram, "helped me get rid of multiple sclerosis."

She gazed out on the surfers riding the waves outside the restaurant window, then with a smile quickly ran her hands down her sides. "Now all I have to do is get rid of some more weight."

With her ruddy face and clear eye, she looked fine for a middle-aged lady from Pasadena who had been through what she had.

Betty Perram laughed good-naturedly. "There is no such thing as getting old unless you make yourself old. And the fastest way to get old is to have emotional problems you can't handle."

Only six months before, she had been without the use of her right leg, hand, and arm, and had no sense of equilibrium. Her nerve ends seemed to be deteriorating.

"The doctor stuck needles in me, and I didn't even feel it."

Her whole world seemed to be collapsing. Her marriage had broken up, she lost her business, and a love affair had gone sour. She began overeating, and put on eighty-five pounds. The jolts were more than her system could bear. She became ill. After a number of tests, San Marino neurologist Louis Duemler advised her she had multiple sclerosis and began treatment with steroids.

Teacher Pat Patrick encouraged her to also use her mind-training. Several times a day she would take the elevator to her mental Workshop.

"I sent a message to every nerve and muscle in my body not to let MS get the best of it. I visualized a purifying process beginning with the skin. I would visually scrub my skin clean, rubbing off the impurities, inside and out. I mentally examined the blood stream, cleansing the corpuscles, then washed off the muscle fibers."

As I listened to her, I couldn't help thinking of a friend, also afflicted with MS, who sat in a wheelchair bemoaning his fate. Both were forty-five years old, but Betty Perram was driven by a will to get well, while he, subconsciously, had hung onto an illness that brought him attention. He would have vehemently denied wanting to stay an invalid, but wouldn't do what Betty Perram had done even when it was shown him he had nothing to lose.

Her doctor had been helpful. "He told me that the will to get better was half the battle, and I just battled overtime."

I had no clear idea how Betty Perram had gotten well. How much of it was the therapy, how much her determination, how much her subconscious visualization? Who was to say? But there was no doubt in Betty Perram's mind what had done it.

In her meditation, she had put herself on a pedestal. "You have to keep building yourself up, countering the blows that toppled you from that pedestal in the first place."

Her mental routine would have done credit to a physical culturist.

"Visually I stretched my muscles, hanging from a steel bar. Mentally I attached sandbags to my feet to add that much more stretch." Her nerve sheaths got special treatment. "I coated my nerves with colored lights, and not knowing which color was most beneficial, I used every color in my imaginary rainbow."

She also went after that eighty-five pounds. She was so fat she found it difficult to love herself, but she felt she had to muster this self-love to get well. So there was nothing to do but lose weight as rapidly as she could, programming a slimming down that would not only make her look better but improve her health as well.

She splashed pictures of bikini-clad girls all over her apartment, including the refrigerator door, which symbolized the doorway to obesity. "I snipped the heads off these shapely figures and, in my levels, put my own head on the bodies. It really did something for my image."

She tried various methods. "I would picture myself sitting scantily garbed under hot floodlights, and see the layers of ugly fat just melting off." She had already lost fifty pounds, and had thirty-five to go.

In six weeks, she noted the improvement in her functioning. Her equilibrium came back, and her impaired right side showed definite movement. Her doctor took a spinal tap and new tests. They were negative. "He told me he had never known anybody to get a remission so quickly."

She told him what she had been doing, and asked if he thought it might have helped.

"He said the mental attitude is a decisive factor in getting well, just as it is in becoming ill."

He took her off ACTH, warning that she would feel depressed until her system readjusted to the "high" the drug had given her.

"I could now sympathize with dope addicts. Withdrawal was a terrible experience."

But Betty had a panacea. She went down into her Community Workshop, where fellow students visualized along with her, and asked for new strength. Almost immediately she felt an excess of energy and had a wonderful feeling of lightness. She had no idea whether this was self-generated or the gift of the others. But she felt the depression lifting like a cloud before the wind. "I was a child of the universe, and the universe was taking care of its own."

There was nothing of the evangelist in Betty Perram. She spoke humbly, grateful that she had been able to turn her life around. "There was something I was meant to learn, and I hope I have learned it."

I found it hard to disagree.

"Isn't it too bad we can't learn these lessons when we're young?"

She smiled easily. "It's never too late. Age is a state of mind, brought on by a feeling of being trapped."

She stretched her arms to the sky and looked out on the gulls skimming low over the beach.

"We have to stay free and open, reaching out constantly, ever meeting new challenges. It makes life worthwhile and keeps you healthy."

She was hopeful of a new relationship and a new job. She had programmed herself for both.

"You only attract people at your own level. And who would be attracted to a big fat slob?"

She climbed into her car to drive the fifty miles to Pasadena.

Her eyes twinkled. "You know, I couldn't have done this a few weeks ago."

Betty Perram called two weeks later to say that she had spoken to her doctor and he would discuss the case with me.

"How do you feel?" I asked.

"Better all the time. I just got through playing a round of golf with the ladies, and I start a new job in three days."

"How about the other?"

"Oh, you mean my love life. I've got another twenty-five or thirty pounds to drop before I get involved again. I'm visualizing perfection these days."

She appeared to hesitate. "You know, through visualization, it came to me that a diet of high protein, low fat, and minimal carbohydrates was good for me, and when I mentioned it to my doctor, he said that some physician in Oregon had already put forward that concept for some cases of MS."

Duemler was inclined to be conservative, but he acknowledged that Betty Perram had been an exceptional patient. She had had MS, and she had recovered. The condition has different degrees of intensity, and Betty's, he said, had not been as severe as some. But there was no question that her attitude (together with the ACTH, of course) had helped. "I have known people with lesser disability than Betty Perram who not only didn't recover but were forced to retire," he said. "They just didn't have her attitude."

Chapter 11

The Other Side

Once the impressionable subconscious was laid open, almost any suggestion at this level could presumably influence the sensitized individual, unless there was a corresponding control. Otherwise, said some, he might very well be subject to the pollution in the minds of others, particularly his instructor. Though I hadn't encountered this myself, I had heard scattered reports of students hallucinating after Alpha-training, and was hardly reassured by an instructor's comment that "they were unbalanced to begin with."

"Many people," cautioned Dr. Elmer Green of the Menninger Clinic in Topeka, "are psychically catapulted into realms in which they cannot protect themselves from dangers arising either from within their own unconscious or from psychic manipulation by other persons. Students are often programmed in ways not appropriate to their own needs, nor at their own proper rates. What is proper for one can be disastrous for another. Many commercial mind-training teachers are incompetent to work with people in matters where psychological and physical health are at stake. Certainly former salesmen who have had a few courses in hypnotic programming are not qualified to work in this very delicate area of the human psyche, with its psychosomatic correlations."

Green, a psychologist, stood almost in horror of the imaginary assistants the student took into his Workshop. "These advisers, however constructed or found," he warned, "may serve as masks for entities to control the student's mental, emotional, and physical behavior."

He had what he considered a clear-cut instance of

demonic possession, observed by a colleague, very much concerned over a couple whose assistants had apparently turned hostile. After Green warned against possession, the distressed pair, taking his advice, sharply challenged their imaginary advisers. A dramatic duel ensued, much like that between the legendary devil and Daniel Webster. Green's friend kept him posted. "The students went down to their Workshops and told their assistants to leave. In both cases, a strong but eventually successful test of wills took place, with the assistants becoming very ugly in the process."

The assistants were presumably no match for the alerted intelligence of the "possessed" husband and wife. Could they have forced them from their minds because of some new awareness, tainted as it was?

How had these assistants manifested their malignancy? How was one to know where the pollution originated? Why had Green's friend become so concerned that he passed on his misgivings to the man from Menninger?

"The wife told me that she had been having increasing trouble getting to sleep at night, or going down to her levels because of hostile and ugly faces in her mind. After her assistants left, she was no longer bothered by the faces; they had disappeared."

The diagnosis of possession had obviously been second-hand. Perhaps Elmer Green had found what he was looking for. However, it seemed quite possible that people with habitually overdrawn imaginations, a hallucinatory drug background, or schizoid tendencies could flip out if their delicate balance was tipped ever so slightly.

All this was a side of the coin I had not experienced. My own Workshop advisers, freely chosen, were professional psychics, and their role had been passive. I had gained little from their presence before dismissing them, and would have discounted Green's warning but for the feeling that perhaps others were more impressionable than myself. However, the advisers could certainly be dispensed with. Or, granting Green's contention, why not then use saints or angels as Workshop consultants? Any sainted adviser could hardly be an evil force, if we were to assume, as did Green, the outside impact on the impressionable subconscious.

"Think good," a teacher had said, "and only good can result."

Green seemed on firm ground with his criticism of unqualified teachers, unprepared personally and professionally, for their sensitive task. He had witnessed some adverse results and received reports on others.

"One of our friends in the Bay Area [San Francisco], a counselor on psychological and religious problems, reported at least a dozen of his clients suffering from paranoid neuroses as a result of taking mind-training courses. A psychiatrist, who took one of the commercial courses himself, reported to us that four of the thirty who went through the program became psychotic. Two of them had to be hospitalized. In part, he attributed this result to the psychic peculiarity of the instructor. Other students with whom we have discussed the 'instructor effect' have reported similarly. Apparently a kind of psychic 'transference' phenomenon can occur—a 'psychic pollution' due to the unconscious receptivity of the subject to the extrasensory perception of the hypnotist."

Green thought of commercial mind-training as hypnosis and the instructors as hypnotists, pointing out the use of hypnosis' traditional countdown system and color progression to engage the focus of the student. Any externally imposed influence over the mind obviously conveyed the unhappy connotation of a Svengali bending an innocent Trilby to his evil will.

"Mind-training teachers often maintain that no harm can be done to another person by themselves or by their students because they are programmed with the idea that if these 'powers' are used for ignoble or selfish persons the powers will be lost. But posthypnotic suggestions are notorious for their impermanence. So if real psychic 'powers' are developed in students, it can be assumed that hypnotically imposed restrictions on the use of such powers will not be long-lasting."

At no time had I had the feeling in my own course of being hypnotized or that I had surrendered any of my volition or control. I felt at all times that I was doing it, and that just as I had a choice of Workshop advisers, so did I have options in pictures and moods into which I visualized myself into Alpha. Counting down twenty-one

134

steps did not make me a creature of Alexander Everett, or of the devil. And wasn't there some form of hypnosis, subliminal to be sure, in almost everything we read in the newspapers or magazines, heard on radio, or watched on television? We were constantly being brainwashed, and if that wasn't hypnosis, it was a pretty fair imitation.

Green did have a kind word for the new world of inner space that commercial mind-training had opened up for so many otherwise confined to the narrow limitations of Beta-thinking. "Hypnotic programming has convinced many people that an inner terrain exists, and in this way, it has been instrumental in drawing attention to an important dimension of human life. But commercialism, even if qualified, should be banished from the Alpha-training field.

"Commercialism often results in exaggerated claims for powers that can be obtained by anyone who pays the price and takes the course, stresses powers not appropriate to certain persons, such as the ability to diagnose and treat diseases, and puts undue emphasis on large enrollment, to earn more money rather than be of service. Large enrollment interferes with one-to-one contact between teachers and students, so that whatever problems arise are unlikely to be properly handled even if the teacher has the proper skill."

Green's conclusions on the risks, or the waste, of unqualified teachers were similar to my own. But I did know of teachers who made up in dedication what they lacked in degrees. Their classes were uniformly small, the contact between students close, and the subsequent study sessions effective. Their fees were frequently elastic.

Green had become involved in mind-training after researching the autogenic training system developed by Dr. Johannes Schultz in Germany. Shortly after the turn of the century, Freud had given up hypnosis as a medical tool because he thought it unpredictable. Schultz was more imaginative. "It occurred to Schultz," said Green, "that perhaps hypnosis was an erratic tool because the patient often unconsciously resisted the doctor. If the patient were able to direct for himself the procedure being used, with the doctor acting as his teacher, then the control technique would come into the realm of self-regulation and perhaps be more effective."

Schultz was interested in making sick people well. If they can think themselves into illness, he reasoned, they should be able to think themselves to health. It was all the same pattern. Through self-suggestion, Schultz found, the individual could quiet his nerves, upgrade his attitude, and gain control over such involuntary functions as respiration and blood flow, even to changing the temperature of various parts of the body at will.

Green combined the self-suggestion technique with modern Biofeedback machines, measuring brainwaves from Alpha through Theta and Delta, muscle-response machines, and temperature-controlling devices. Teamed with his wife, Alyce, and associate Dale Walters, he came upon a powerful therapeutic tool. "If a person's heart is malfunctioning from psychosomatic causes, it is certainly not 'all in his head,' but knowing that the cause is psychosomatic does not tell him what he can do about it. When his heart rate is displayed on a meter, however, he can easily and objectively experiment with the psychological states that influence the rate."

Green's training methods were elementary in their simplicity. Autogenic, self-suggestive phrases were used to induce relaxation—"be calm and quiet." There was brainwave feedback for self-information, and deep-breathing techniques taught by the Yogi Swami Rama. "The breathing exercises included hyperventilation, to activate the central nervous system, followed by slow, even breathing for quieting the body and mind and for focusing attention. We used auditory signals for brainwave feedback, different tones signifying the presence of different brainwaves, a low tone for Theta, a higher tone for Alpha."

Hooked up with Biofeedback machines to measure brainwaves, skin temperature, and muscle response, subjects sat in comfortable chairs in a quiet, dimly lit room, so different from the glaring lights of my own classroom. For fifteen minutes, the EEG (electroencephalograph) measured Alpha and Theta feedback, then Theta alone for a half hour. Furnished portable brainwave feedback machines, students practiced an hour a day, recording their visual experiences together with Alpha-Theta duration levels.

From research with housewives and college students, Green had made an interesting Biofeedback discovery. "While using any kind of Biofeedback device for learning something about yourself, it is interesting and instructive to experimentally induce in yourself a feeling of anxiety and nervousness, then calmness and tranquility. You can play with anger and with peacefulness, then you can experiment with muscle tension, relaxation, slow deep-breathing, learning to manipulate processes while seeing the meter."

The Greens trained a group of housewives to increase the temperature of their hands, using an adaptation of Schultz's autogenic training. They had variable results. Next, using autogenic training and Biofeedback machines, they attempted to train eighteen college students to control muscle tension in the right forearm, temperature of a finger on the right hand, and an Alpha brainwave pattern. Muscle response was picked up from a myograph electrode attached with salt paste to the skin, the temperature obtained from a thermistor taped to the middle finger, and brainwave signals on the electroencephalograph from an electrode attached to the left occiput, or the part of the brain governing involuntary functions.

A subject's hand, responding to self-suggestion, usually of a visual nature, would sometimes show a temperature change of ten degrees, reflecting an accelerated flow of blood to the area. Deliberate thinking, Beta-thinking, of course, worked against the desired end. "If a subject tried to force the temperature to rise by active volition," Green found, "it invariably went down. But if he relaxed, 'told the body' what to do, and then detached himself from the response, the temperature would rise.

"Quite often with beginners the hand temperature will rise at first, but then an insidious thought will creep in, such as, 'It may work with other people, but it probably won't work for me.' This precipitates vasoconstriction of the sympathetic nervous system, and blood flow in the hands is appropriately reduced. Within a few seconds, temperature of the hands begins to drop."

With the EEG, the Greens were able to correlate

categorically certain brainwave patterns with specific thought and behavior processes. "When people focus attention on the outside world, they usually produce only Beta frequencies. If they close their eyes and think of nothing in particular, they generally produce a mixture of Alpha and Beta. If they slip toward sleep, become drowsy, Theta frequencies often appear and there is less of Alpha and Beta. Delta waves were not normally present except in deep sleep."

The Greens noted that the state associated with Theta contained very clear imagery. "Pictures or ideas would spring full-blown into consciousness without the person being aware of their creation. The Theta reverie, as we began to call it, was definitely different from a daydreaming state, and much to our surprise, it seemed to correspond with descriptions given by geniuses of the past of the state of consciousness they experienced while being their most creative."

Obviously the Greens had come upon a condition which commercial mind-trainers were already emulating, suggesting any visualization which they felt induced Alpha in their subjects, but which apparently also induced a mixture of Theta as well. This explained perhaps why Lennie Weitz, asleep, was the star of our Alpha class. With his conscious mind completely turned off, his eyes constantly closed, he may very well have been in the slower, more creative Theta rhythm. We would never know for sure, not having used the Biofeedback machines with their auditory as well as visual signal system.

Some results reported by the Greens paralleled the output by students in my Alpha class. Despite Green's feeling that his subjects were autogenically trained, while commercial students were under some hypnotic spell, there seemed little difference in the way mind changes took place. "After only a week or two of Alpha and Theta practice, several students reported a change in their dreams. Not only were they able to recall more of their dreams, but their dreams became much more vivid and meaningful. After three or four weeks, they began reporting subjective impressions, which, while hardly earth-shaking, were important to them.

" 'I feel so good after a session, so much more confident. I feel like whatever I have to do I can do.' Or, 'I feel so with it,' or, 'I feel so put together.'

" 'It makes me feel fearless, like I could conquer the world. The only way I can describe it is to use the word *elated.*'

" 'I've really changed somehow inside, and other people can feel it. When I walk down the halls at school, people that I meet who I don't even know say, "Hi, how are you doing?" ' "

Students reported an increased perceptiveness and an increased sense of responsiblity with this perceptiveness. Some were more tolerant of their fellows and better able to work with them. Family relationships eased. There were rewards in schoolwork. Better concentration, less tension, and less fatigue.

"I had this zoology test coming up; I studied all night. Then I practiced Alpha-Theta from nine-thirty to ten-thirty and had my test at eleven. I'd been up all night, and yet I was able to relax and I did just fine."

The same student gathered volumes of information for a written paper, and then seemed to have forgotten everything he'd read. In his Alpha-Theta session, he became very relaxed, and his mind began drifting lazily through the mass of information he had assimilated until it all fell together.

Other students relived experiences with a vividness they had not known originally, even to sounds, tastes, and smells. It was almost as if they could reach out for all the yesterdays they had not fully savored at the time.

"I began first just sort of thinking of a bicycle I wanted to buy. And then I thought about the bicycle I had when I was a kid. And then, zap, I was back in my childhood, into a whole set of childhood feelings connected with sounds and smells, how the gate grated, all kinds of things. The smell of the backyard, of the whole neighborhood. I was just totally lost for a while in this experience. It wasn't like just remembering what the backyard looked like, but the smells and the sounds. That was new and different."

The visual experiences of some Green students clearly bordered on the psychic. Unbidden images of going through a dark narrow tunnel (being born, perhaps), or through a tunnel seeing a light or sunset at its end. "Images of climbing downstairs, or upstairs, images of a cave or pyramid, all very realistic experiences." Some saw an eye—a single eye—perhaps the third eye of psychic symbolism? "Several had images of a teacher or a guide, the wise old man [were they subconsciously reaching out for assistants?]. And several had images of a book of knowledge that held special information for them. Sometimes it was held by a professor, a doctor, or a librarian." Again, were they involuntarily invoking the advisers that Green's methodology denied them?

From research with autogenic training, and with a Yoga adept, such as the Swami Rama, the Greens felt that any physiological process objectively discerned by the subject could be self-controlled to some degree. "Blood pressure, blood flow, heart rate, lymph flow, muscle tension, brainwaves, all these have already been self-regulated through training in one laboratory or another."

Green projected this self-mastery to the individual beneficially managing his own health and well-being. "If every young student knew by the time he finished his first biology class in grade school that the body responds to self-generated psychological inputs, that blood flow and heart behavior, as well as a host of other body processes, can be influenced at will, it would change prevailing ideas about both physical and mental health. It would then be quite clear and understandable that we are individually responsible to a large extent for our state of health or disease."

In a very real sense, he saw us as masters of our own fate. "Perhaps then people would begin to realize that it is not life that kills us but rather our reaction to it, and this reaction can be to a significant extent self-chosen."

In the Swami Rama, of Rishikesh and the Himalayas, the Greens had a supreme example of the ultimate in autogenic training. At Menninger's, under laboratory conditions, the Swami Rama demonstrated his isolated control over the circulation to his hands and, incredibly, stopped his heart for seventeen seconds. "We had wired him for brainwaves, respiration, skin potential, skin resistance, heart behavior (EKG), blood flow in his hands, and body temperature."

Ironically, the Swami was called upon to prove in the laboratory a natural power flowing freely out of man's union with the universe. It was the triumph of a clear channel over the static of the machines. "While thus encumbered," said Green, "the Swami caused two areas a couple of inches apart on the palm of his right hand to gradually change temperature in opposite directions, at a maximum rate of about four degrees Fahrenheit per minute, until they showed a temperature difference of about ten degrees. The left side of his palm, totally motionless through this performance, looked as if it had been slapped with a ruler a few times; it was rosy red. The right side of his hand had turned ashen gray."

Almost instantaneously the Swami jumped his heart rate from seventy beats to three hundred beats per minute, precipitating an "atrial flutter," in which the heart fired at its maximum rate without blood filling the chambers properly or the valves performing normally. "In effect, the Swami stopped his heart from pumping blood for at least seventeen seconds, this being his technique for obliterating his pulse during examination by medical doctors."

The Swami, of course, was no average man. He made Alpha, Theta, and Delta brainwaves at will, even though Delta had never before been recorded in anything but a deep-sleep pattern. And while apparently sleeping, even snoring at times, he still remembered everything said in the room during twenty-five minutes of testing. He was another Lennie Weitz.

The Swami's accomplishments showed there were almost no boundaries to what the gifted individual could achieve with proper training. "The Swami," observed an impressed Green, "could diagnose physical ailments very much in the manner of Edgar Cayce [the Virginia Beach mystic], except that he appeared to be totally conscious, though with indrawn attention for a few seconds, while he was 'picking up' information." He could also call off, correctly, the titles in a stranger's library.

I wondered what the scientifically oriented Green would have thought of Cathy Francis diagnosing stomach cancer, John Burnham tuning into pelvic disorder, or Dorothy Nelson attempting to dissolve the cataracts of a half-blind woman. Without knowing quite how it was done, I suspected they were all tuned into frequencies which we were as yet incapable of isolating.

The experiments with the Swami revealed that a brain-wave mixture was not only normal but apparently essential for maximum results. "When the Swami produced Alpha, he did not cease the production of Beta. And when he produced Theta, both Alpha and Beta were retained about fifty percent of the time. Likewise, when he produced Delta, he was also producing Theta, Alpha, and Beta a relatively high percentage of the time. Perhaps this tells us something important. If one wishes to be aware of the hypnagogic [drowsy-state] imagery associated with Theta, it may be necessary to retain Alpha since it is a conscious state when Theta is produced."

As the Swami had so dramatically shown, mind and body are sufficiently related to be one. There is no real distinction, and what affects one plane affects the other. "Every change in the physiological state is accompanied by an appropriate change in the mental-emotional state, conscious or unconscious, and conversely, every change in the mental-emotional state, conscious or unconscious, is accompanied by an appropriate change in the physiological state."

There was nothing magic about what was taking place when a subject fired brainwaves. One part or hemisphere of the brain, the cerebral cortex, featured Beta or conscious thought, and its cranio-spinal nervous system controlled the voluntary muscular system. The unconscious side, controlling the subconscious mind, contained the subcortical brain, the old lower brain structure that man shares with most mammals, and the autonomic or involuntary nervous system, controlling the skin, internal organs, and the circulatory system.

The old brain, the paleocortex, included the visceral brain, involved in psychosomatic regulation. And so in affecting this area of the brain, the individual influenced and modified his health and behavior to a striking extent. "It's quite clear from recent research that electrical stimulation of the visceral brain and related neural structures through implanted electrodes caused emotional changes in humans. Conversely, perceptual and emotional changes are followed by neural changes or responses."

Ironically, Green and Alexander didn't seem too far apart in outlook. Green spoke of Theta when we, machineless, spoke of Alpha. He spoke of reverie when we spoke of imagery and visualization. Almost poetically, recalling Alexander's grandiosity, Green heralded what the new awareness could do for mankind. "The entrance or key to all these inner processes, we are beginning to believe, is a particular state of consciousness to which we have given the undifferentiated name 'reverie.' This reverie can be approached by Theta brainwave-training [how about the Alpha mix?], in which the gap between conscious and unconscious processes is voluntarily narrowed, and even temporarily eliminated. When that self-regulated reverie is established, the body can apparently be programmed at will and the instructions carried out. Emotional states can be dispassionately examined, accepted or rejected, or totally supplanted by others deemed more useful, and problems insoluble in the normal state of consciousness can be elegantly resolved."

Green had more vision than most scientists. "It seems increasingly certain," he said in a brilliant burst of insight, "that healing and creativity are different pieces of a single picture." The Swami Rama maintained that self-healing could be performed in a state of creative reverie, the images for giving the body instructions manipulated in a manner similar to that in which ideas are creatively handled for the solution of intellectual problems, not by deduction, but by a flash of intuition from the subconscious. "Creativity in terms of physiological processes means then physical healing, physical regeneration. Creativity in emotional terms consists then of establishing or creating attitude changes through the practice of healthful emotions, emotions that establish in the visceral brain those neurological patterns whose reflection in the viscera is one that physicians approve as a stress resistant."

As thorough as he was in his own domain, psychologist Green could only suggest the tremendous scope of brainwave therapy. A physician, perhaps a psychiatrist, who recognized the psychosomatic nature of man's ills, was needed to execute, and perhaps validate, everything we knew about Alpha-Theta training and Biofeedback.

"It would seem," observed Green, "that brainwave-

143

training could be helpful in all forms of psychotherapy, since it provides a way for patients to vividly experience, or reexperience, through imagery in Theta reverie, normally unconscious material. This material, physical, emotional, or mental, could be brought into consciousness quite easily and handled, with the help of a therapist, in a creative way."

It was indeed an enlightened suggestion. All it needed was a psychiatrist who considered mind and body as one and was sufficiently dedicated to use whatever tools were available to help his sick.

Chapter 12

A Pragmatic Look

John Balog was a psychiatrist, but first and foremost, he was a physician dedicated to helping the sick.

"Fundamentally," said Dr. Balog, "the average person heals himself, and as he relaxes in Alpha, healing is accelerated and the body normalized."

We were in a Pasadena restaurant, not far from his office, as the doctor casually discussed powers of the mind ordinarily espoused by some East Indian guru. In an adjacent booth, I could pick out two old ladies from Pasadena, and beyond them a trio of giggling postdebs—certainly as prosaic a scene as you could imagine.

The doctor followed my glance and smiled. "There is nothing esoteric about Biofeedback. We are exploring the hidden potential of the mind and getting the patient to use it for his own good."

At forty, Balog was obviously a new breed of psychiatrist, a physician not only involved in healing the mind but in using that mind to heal the body. As yet, it was all so new that the therapists were learning along with the patients.

Even before his interest in Biofeedback, he had adapted the progressive-relaxation technique of a distinguished psychotherapist and found it useful in taking some mental patients off medication. As medical director of the Mental Health Unit of Glendale Adventist Hospital, he had become concerned by the amount of tranquilizers people were taking and the consequent abuse, indicating the ineffectiveness, to some degree, of traditional psychotherapy. "I saw the shortcomings of the conventional therapy in people taking so long to get to know about their own feelings. Sometimes it took years of psycho-analysis for people to know themselves, and so often it never happened at all."

His results with progressive relaxation were mixed, and then with the appearance of Biofeedback machines, he immediately saw their potential. "We now had a definite way," he pointed out, "to measure the state of relaxation and reproduce it on demand."

Essentially conservative, like most doctors, he was still open enough to use any technique that worked. Despite his relative youth, he was a serious-faced man, with a warm smile that suddenly made him look boyishly younger. His credentials were solidly conventional. He had his medical degree from the University of Michigan, and had taken resident training at UCLA. He spoke plainly, seldom using medical terms, and never mentioned his patients by name, though I got the impression they all had their special identities as far as he was concerned. He was less than middle height, and slight, but he gave the impression of an imposing substantiality and calm.

He had delved thoroughly into the pioneer work of the neural psychiatrist Johannes Schultz of Germany, and had pointed to the rows of newly published volumes dealing with Schultz's work in autogenic training with a variety of ailments and situations, from easing the horrors of the dental chair to refraining from wetting the bed nights.

"Schultz," he now observed, "would condition his people by telling them they were to feel heavier and warmer. It was the simplest inductive process, but in responding to this suggestion, patients eventually relaxed sufficiently to normalize their bodies and begin the healing process."

In the Biofeedback area, he worked closely with his psychologist wife, Dawn, and left the testing in her capable hands. When psychotherapy was indicated, before, during, or subsequent to the Biofeedback sessions, he proceeded with due consideration to the information conveyed by the individual's tested response to the machines.

However, the machines had more often than not served as a shortcut in actual therapy and, in some cases, produced surprising results, demonstrating how readily the ailing could heal themselves.

Looking around the restaurant, in the most casual manner, the doctor observed with a wave of the hand, "We discovered for instance, that by increasing the circulation to the fingers we eliminated migraine headaches."

He had been treating a patient for a narrowing of the capillaries in the fingers, with the suggestion that he visualize anything that would bring blood to them.

The patient, who had a history of migraine, visualized his hand in a warm tub.

"Not only was there a temperature rise of several degrees in the patient's hand but the circulation to the head was noticeably increased. We could actually see the sudden pulse of blood in the temple and the headache would disappear."

All the patient had to do, thereafter, was to mentally put his hand in warm water, and the headaches would leave. And in time, as inner relaxation became a pattern, they disappeared completely.

Unlike many self-styled scientific researchers, Dr. Balog not only tested others but practiced on the machines himself. He had varied the temperature of his hand several degrees, both raising and lowering the temperature sensor with his own thoughts, and had similarly activated the electromyograph with the electrical stimulus from visualizing his own muscle movements.

He practiced with the electroencephalograph regularly, producing Alpha at will, as he found this quickened his awareness and better enabled him to tune into his patients. He checked over Biofeedback training of patients at a Glendale hospital, finding that the meditation appeared to hasten their recovery time.

Because of his own familiarity with the machines, he realized how Biofeedback helped people to dramatically understand the relationship of their bodies and minds. "It is amazing how little people know about what is happening to them physically and mentally, or how little control the average person has over functions on which his very existence depends."

What Green established experimentally, Balog applied pragmatically. "In Alpha-Theta, the individual can learn to manage his blood pressure, raise or lower the temperature of various parts of his body, contract or dilate his blood vessels, and even control nerve impulses to his muscles. We have one Biofeedback patient who regained use of a partially paralyzed arm, and another who conquered Raynaud's Phenomenon, a circulatory disorder marked by pain and spasms in the fingers and toes, which can lead to gangrene."

In the case of the disabled arm, the Alpha-trained patient had been hooked up, additionally, to an electromyograph, measuring his muscle response in Alpha, and had gradually learned to establish muscle movement by visualizing the desired muscle response.

"In Raynaud's Phenomenon," said Balog, "a temperature sensor machine was attached to the patient's arm and the suggestion was made that he increase the temperature to his fingers, expanding the constricted blood vessels in the fingers."

"You mean," I said, "that by just sending thoughts in Alpha to his fingers the blood vessels responded in a healing way?"

"Actually what he did was to normalize the function of those blood vessels, and normalization is what healing is all about."

Certain alternatives suggested themselves. "Couldn't the patient have increased circulation to his fingers with exercise?"

"That would bring blood to the extremities, just as dipping the hands in hot water would. But the effect would only be temporary and not reach the seat of the problem. By getting the brain to send the impulse to dilate the blood vessels, you may be reversing the process that brought on the dysfunction in the first place. Some therapists feel that eighty percent of human illness is of psychogenic origin, and so getting at the source, you are better able to treat the disorder."

I had observed psychic healers reach out with their own minds and apparently transmit a healing vibration to an impressionable subject, and it had made me wonder whether there might not be a healing frequency in the atmosphere, just as there were different radio and television frequencies.

Balog shrugged. "The individual has the power in his own mind to heal himself, by establishing contact with his own body and mind. Additionally the concept of self-healing gives the individual the needed confidence to be well, and stay well, in the process of mastering his own functions."

He didn't think of his Biofeedback cases in terms of cures, but as improvements, even when they were apparently cured. "Self-improvement is the crux of the problem, trying to improve ourselves through self-knowledge. We have to know where we are to know where we're going."

There had been progress in every case. "Even with a diabetic, treated primarily for tension, the patient's insulin intake was noticeably decreased. He is learning how to relax inwardly for the first time in his life, and it's normalizing his body functions."

Was it all as simple as relaxation?

"It is a deeper relaxation, below the conscious Beta level. For instance, the patient with the paralyzed arm was asked to visualize whatever would help him move the muscle. He pictured a lever, a crane, a pulley, another arm, each moving that muscle for him. It didn't matter what he visualized, as long as it represented effective outside help to him."

I was reminded of the similarity to my own Alpha-schooling in visualization.

He listened politely. "How did you know you were in Alpha?"

"I seemed to be more in tune with people and what they were thinking."

Without the Biofeedback, my Alpha was obviously totally subjective, and yet he did not question me as one skeptical student had questioned a rather overbearing instructor.

"How do I know I'm in Alpha?" the student had asked.

"You're in Alpha," this worthy replied, "when I tell you you're in Alpha."

Balog laughed along with me.

His interest in Alpha was purely remedial—and preventive. If visualization and meditation could get people well, why wouldn't it keep them well, averting the agony and expense of unnecessary illness?

"Doctors should make themselves aware of what benefits the patient and use it as long as it works. I observed

149

Alpha Biofeedback sufficiently in the laboratory to recognize its deep, relaxing influence, knowing that the patient improves readily while free of internal conflict and worsens with it."

Some psychologists had cautioned against emotionally unstable persons producing Alpha. He didn't categorically agree. "I wouldn't encourage any further imagination by schizophrenics, already afflicted with an excess of imagination. But anybody who can distinguish reality from unreality should be able to use Alpha safely."

Others had warned Biofeedback-training could be harmful to drug users.

An amused glint came to the physician's eyes. "Well, it could normalize their body functions, so they would be achieving some satisfactory state of pleasure without drugs. It could ease their insomnia and help them relax, and give them a high feeling of elation without stimulants. It is a non-drug way of establishing contact with the body." He smiled. "If all this is harmful, then it can harm them."

Some reactions in Alpha were totally unpredictable. Contrary to expectation, a thirty-nine-year-old woman treated for alcoholism constantly registered Alpha when she became angry instead of the Beta normally reflecting an emotional state.

In resolving the paradox, Balog added to the lore of an infant field. "Feeling put upon by her husband, she needed the excuse of being drunk to express her normally suppressed anger without guilt. In reliving the situation with Biofeedback, she threw off the guilt, resulting in a deep sense of relaxation as she released herself emotionally for the first time, sober."

The implication was startling. It was not emotion that crippled an individual but the internal conflict it reflected. The anger that produced Alpha was obviously of a different nature from that reflected in Beta brainwaves. Beta anger was nonproductive, even counterproductive; Alpha anger, on the other hand, apparently induced a mental state in which the individual liberated himself.

"Essentially," said Balog, "it's a question of self-mastery. Nobody can be in constant conflict with himself and be productive and healthy."

Had the woman actually healed herself?

"In Alpha, this patient recognized her destructive pattern of behavior, and it led to her awakening. But of course, she has to keep meditating to keep from reverting."

She had stayed away from alcohol for almost a year, except for one lapse, when she quarreled with her husband over his drinking. "She began drinking to stand up to him. But in her new awareness, she quickly recognized what she had done, and it didn't happen again."

As a rule, only patients unresponsive to conventional therapy were put on Biofeedback, guided by the doctor's wife, a clinical psychologist, who had done clinical research in brainwaves.

They used three different machines: the electroencephalograph (EEG), to measure Alpha and Theta brainwaves; the electromyograph (EMG), reflecting specific muscle response to mind activity; and a thermistor, which recorded the rise in body heat wherever it was attached.

"Contrary to popular opinion, Biofeedback machines don't produce Alpha or Theta brainwaves. The individual makes the waves. The EEG machine indicates at what point he's producing Alpha, so that he may repeat this thinking and reproduce these brainwaves at will.

"We discovered that a patient heals rapidly in the slower, relaxing Alpha-Theta brainwave cycles, which are so often evident in restful sleep. We get the patient to produce these cycles, first with the machines, and after a while without the machines. With practice, the individual generally knows when he's in Alpha from the way he feels."

One didn't have to be a superman to get results. "Just by closing his eyes the average person can produce up to eighty percent of Alpha, and perhaps some Theta, requiring the elimination of a twenty-percent Beta factor, which works against the deep relaxation required for self-healing."

His Biofeedback candidates were usually prone to anxiety states, hypertension, migraine, and other tension syndromes. Even so, each case was different and had to be analyzed separately.

"You don't take away symptoms without giving some

advantage in return. Otherwise the subject will revert to his original symptoms."

With Biofeedback temperature-training, controlling the blood flow, a woman with a migraine history got rid of her headaches in three sessions. But in doing so, she lost the "advantage" they had given her for years in controlling her husband and children.

"When she no longer panicked them into doing what she wanted for fear of bringing on these headaches, she went right back to the headaches. People first have to see for themselves how they invite illnesses. Then they're more likely to give up the advantages of their symptoms." He frowned a moment. "Instead of mastering herself, this woman chose to master her family."

Without the desire to change, the most positive Biofeedback results could be little more than a routine exercise.

Balog looked up with a smile.

"Have you ever heard of the Biofeedback athlete?"

I shook my head.

"He makes all the machines respond perfectly. He complains of a backache, and with the EMG attached to his back, he brings the needle down to the desired point. With a history of headaches, he is able to increase his hand temperature at will, and he performs spectacularly on the EEG, producing showers of Alpha without any difficulty. But none of this does anything for him because he's preprogrammed. He's already told himself that the mastery of these machines has nothing to do with his life style of his symptoms. 'Just because I control the machines,' he tells himself, 'it doesn't mean it will help.'"

"Why then," I asked, "does he bother with all these tests?"

"To prove that they can't help him. That's why a patient has to be shown some advantage in changing."

He removed symptoms and medicines gradually. "Beginners stay on their medicines for a while, gradually reducing them as they get used to the idea of getting better. With deep relaxation, the metabolism frequently changes, and the medicine requirement changes with it. We slowly take people with sleep problems off barbiturates, as they find with reduced tension they can sleep naturally."

In the case of a diabetic, trying only to lower tension with Alpha, a metabolism change resulted in an unexpected reduction in insulin. "With adults in turmoil, blood sugar fluctuates widely. Once the emotional state is stabilized, insulin requirements become more predictable."

The new mind-mastery had to be continually reinforced. "Six-month follow-ups have shown that where patients didn't continue with the program, symptoms invariably returned."

Tension was a syndrome of modern living. Truck drivers, plumbers, laborers were as much affected as intellectual writers, artists, teachers, lawyers. It was a rising factor in heart disease, high blood pressure (hypertension), ulcers, and countless other symptoms, such as arthritis, often masked as something else.

As a by-product of tension, high blood pressure was particularly susceptible to deep relaxation. By changing the body's response to tension, pressure could be appreciably lowered. "Often doctors can talk soothingly to a patient and the blood pressure will promptly go down. But the object is to get the patient to reduce his tension through literally talking to himself."

In his pragmatic way, Balog differed with the pedants who wanted to keep Alpha-training a laboratory tool. "Let us put it in the high schools, in health education, letting young people learn they have control over both the voluntary and involuntary functions of their body. Our questing youth don't have to learn mysterious Eastern mantras to gain mastery over their minds and bodies. Simple Alpha-training will give them a healthy high and help them understand themselves."

I had been through several mind-training courses without showing any sign of the genius Alexander had held out for me. Perhaps it was because I no longer troubled to go into my Workshop or meditate unless I had some specific problem.

"You should go through the Biofeedback experience," Balog said with a challenging smile.

"I've had my Alpha-training."

"You're not quite sure you were in Alpha, or what put you there."

I was sure my visualization had done it, developing my memory and the creative faculty as well, through constantly exercising the imagination.

"In learning to control the machines," he said, "you know when you are controlling your own mind."

"But I have nothing wrong with me."

"Not that you know of."

"Well, I could sleep better, I suppose, calm down, get rid of that queasy stomach, and write with greater ease."

"Is that all?" He grinned. "I'll tell Dawn you'll be in for your Biofeedback-training."

"If there's anything to the courses I took, I should be able to produce Alpha at will."

He shrugged. "Who knows? You might be a Biofeedback athlete."

Chapter 13

Science, Science!

I was now part of a scientific experience. I sat expectantly as Dawn slipped the electrodes of the electroencephalograph onto the side of my head, parting the hair to establish contact with my scalp over the brain area and applying a special paste designed to accelerate this contact.

Before me there was a narrow panel of eight lights, and to my left a machine, manned by Dawn, which recorded on tape the number and nature of my Alpha brainwaves as I spoke, meditated, thought, or in any other way invoked the faculties of my mind.

I looked appreciatively at Dawn, enjoying the feeling of being fussed over by somebody so attractive. I felt myself insensibly drifting off, relaxing much as I would in the barber's chair before a shave.

"In the relaxed state," said Dawn, "the Alpha waves are usually prominent."

"How will I know I'm in Alpha?"

"The panel in front of you will light up."

"Has this anything to do itself with producing Alpha?"

"I'm not so sure. Originally I thought of the Biofeedback machine only as an electronic yardstick, but people perceiving their own Alpha output seem in time to turn it off and on at will."

"In other words, they relate Alpha to whatever sensations they had at the time."

She nodded. "Generally, in Alpha, the individual experiences a feeling of well-being and has a sharpened awareness of his own thoughts and sensations."

I mentioned having gone into my levels and feeling a

broader dimension of the mind. "Couldn't I tell I was in Alpha by my increased awareness?"

"It would still be unscientific—without the machine."

With Biofeedback, progress in producing Alpha was accelerated. The Alpha activity was frequently doubled in the second session and tripled in the third, reaffirming the value of being able to associate internal feelings with an externally perceived barometer.

"Does everybody give off the same Alpha?" I asked.

Dawn laughed good-naturedly.

"Does everybody play the violin or write as well? It varies with the potential."

"You are then into the subconscious state?"

"You can call it that if you like, but it doesn't seem to have the same well-defined boundaries as the conscious —sensory—mind."

For the sake of semantics, I had long before accepted the view that the dream, deep-memory, hypnotic states, and the phase of intuitive awareness, the so-called unconscious faculties, were functions of the subconscious mind and reflective of Alpha or Theta brainwaves.

"By and large," I said, "does every individual produce Alpha?"

She shook her head. "We've noticed that adolescents with behavioral problems or young people on drugs—marijuana, for instance—seem to have difficulty producing Alpha. They may go through a whole session without putting on one light."

Having researched drugs thoroughly, I had not been able to escape the conclusion that marijuana—the good old pot that so many were trying to legalize—distorted the mind and dwindled its capacity to make selective judgments. Now it was apparent that such drugs, as well as the barbiturates and tranquilizers, sold in tons over drugstore counters, had a tendency to block off production of extradimensional Alpha, with its potential for creating and healing.

It brought up an interesting point.

"If you induce Alpha activity where there was little or none before, does that signify that a drug or behavioral problem is being helped?"

Dawn had no glib answer.

"Hopefully," she said, "just as we discovered therapeutic values of Alpha in migraine headaches, hypertension, high blood pressure, and the like."

Obviously people weren't consulting a medical doctor to provide research material for the scientists or to improve their awareness. They were presumably looking for help on a broader front.

"They usually have some problem they want to correct," Dawn said. "It may be something psychosomatic, physical, mental, spiritual. Or they just aren't happy with themselves and the way their lives are going."

She gave a gasp of satisfaction as she completed the job of hooking me up to the electroencephalograph.

"You're ready to function," she said.

I checked the panel.

One or two red lights lit up, then quickly flickered out.

"What does that mean?"

"That was your Alpha output at the moment."

I closed my eyes and meditated, trying to visualize the sea outside my front door—my passive scene from nature.

"I'll bet it's lighting up now."

"No"—she hesitated—"one or two lights flashing on and off."

It occurred to me that the lighting up of the board was in itself eventful.

"What, actually, is putting those lights on?"

She smiled. "You are, with the electrical energy from your brain."

"You mean that I am actually producing electricity?"

She nodded. "And as you continue to test yourself, turning on Alpha at will, your electrical output will increase."

"Is there any limit to this electrical capacity?"

"It's a matter of development. You have billions of brain cells, and each has an energy pattern. The possibilities are endless."

As I considered her remarks, visualizing my brain as a vast dynamo, I glanced up at the panel and saw all eight buttons brightly lit up.

"Isn't this a little strange, for the board to light up with Alpha when I'm consciously concentrating on our conversation?"

A slight frown had wrinkled her forehead. "Normally," she said, "Alpha waves vanish with mental activity requiring attention and visual movement."

"Then why would I be producing Alpha?"

She thought a moment. "As a professional interviewer, you are probably thoroughly relaxed asking questions. And since you don't take notes, deep-memory patterns may very well be alerted in the process."

"And the memory," I finished, "is a function of the Alpha mind."

"Your subconscious mind may be working like a computer—analyzing, sorting, and dissecting the material the conscious mind is receiving."

Obviously something of a subconscious nature was going on. For every time I became absorbed in our conversation, the red lights would flash on in unison. Yet, when I tried to meditate, my mind wandered, conscious of this effort, and the lights would blink off.

Dawn recalled that where the stimulation was not unusual a reaction of alert attention, usually a Beta response, was often accompanied by Alpha. "If you were a bricklayer asking questions in this area," she elaborated, "you would undoubtedly be in Beta. But since it is no novelty for you to be probing into the metaphysical, you are clearly under no effort."

It somehow threw me off to think that I was giving off Beta while meditating and Alpha while apparently going through a rational thought process.

"I don't seem to be getting anywhere."

She laughed. "You're giving off more Alpha than anybody I've seen yet."

"But I have no idea what it means."

"You have to set goals, and then you will see progress."

"What goals?"

"Anything you would like to achieve."

"Writing a revealing novel about the mysteries of life, for instance?"

"Yes, that would be a legitimate goal."

"How about a good marriage?"

She nodded. "That begins with you, so that also would be legitimate, as we all know one has to be ready for marriage."

Her reasoning seemed valid. But what did it have to do with lighting up a lot of red lights?

"You forget," she said, "that's only the measuring rod. It's what the lights reflect that counts."

"And what do they reflect?"

"The altered state of awareness that will make possible the aims you are willing to work for."

In the hour together, one thing had become apparent. My earlier training had made it easier for me to think Alpha, and yet I could very well be one of Balog's Biofeedback athletes. I could produce vast amounts of Alpha and still not accomplish anything unless I related it meaningfully to the course of my life.

I had ample time to consider my introduction to Biofeedback. There had been no breath-taking revelations, I had not fixed on any universal truths, and I had no clearer grasp of my own little problems.

Dawn didn't share my misgivings. "Rome wasn't built in a day," she said cheerfully, as she deftly adjusted the EEG for the second session. "Even in questioning yourself, it shows you're taking stock of yourself. That's a necessary preliminary to understanding."

She turned to the EEG machine and showed me a narrow roll of paper about twice as wide as a stockmarket tape. I saw a close succession of steep slanted lines, some spiking abruptly higher than the others. These, she explained, were Alpha cycles of greater amplitude—part of my first day's output.

As before, the Alpha panel lit up when I questioned Dawn closely. I found this distracting, as I was eager to learn whether I could light up Alpha by simulating the meditative states in my own Alpha-training.

I had had several minor psychic experiences and wondered whether I could relate them to Alpha.

Dawn regarded me curiously. "What kind of experience?"

I thought back to younger days. "I played some poker with other newspapermen, and would invariably know when my first two cards were aces, even though the second card was dealt face down."

She seemed suddenly intrigued. "How could you tell?"

"I would feel a tingle in my stomach, akin, in Yoga, to

the onset of Kundalini, the invisible spiral presumably responsible for arousing the latent powers of the mind."

She was understandably confused. "That's a lot of power for a card game."

"The stakes were steep, and my salary small."

She knew nothing of poker. "But how was this knowledge significant?"

"In five-card stud poker, with three cards still to be dealt, it gave me a distinct betting advantage. A pair of aces was normally a winning hand, but I would bet the pair blind, as they say, not looking at my hole card, and everybody bet along with me, not thinking I had anything more than an ace-high hand."

"But wouldn't they have suspected you had two aces by the way you were betting?"

"Not when I continued to bet without looking at the face-down card."

"But wasn't this taking unfair advantage?"

"If I had been wrong, I would have paid for it."

"But you weren't wrong?"

"I could have still been outdrawn."

"But your intuitive flash or hunch gave you the edge."

"Exactly," I said. "Isn't that what intuition is supposed to do?"

She still wasn't quite sure. "Well, if you put it that way."

"Isn't that what we're trying to do, gain an advantage in life with this Alpha awareness?"

"Not to the disadvantage of others."

The discussion had gotten away from the simple experiment I had visualized. "All I wanted to know was whether I might have been in Alpha when I felt this tingling sensation."

She eyed me brightly. "Perhaps, if you tried to recapture the subjective feeling you had at the time, you might be able to repeat the brainwave activity."

"How am I going to get my stomach to tingle?"

"Just imagine something that will bring on that feeling, remember one of the games and play it back in your mind."

"As simple as that?"

"That's the value of Biofeedback. It lets you know how

much Alpha you are producing when you are thinking or feeling a certain way."

I tried to think of the poker game, and visualized my opponents around the table—their faces became clear and sharp. I renewed the long past picture of an open ace being served to me across the table, then another face down. There was almost a conditioned response, like a Pavlovian reflex. I felt an instant tingle in the pit of my stomach. My eyes turned to the panel of lights. All eight were lit up.

Dawn's eyes followed mine. "You must have done something right."

Again I tried meditating, imagining the rolling surf in front of my home, and again one or two red lights quickly flashed on and off. Everything seemed turned around. Here I was freely spawning Alpha when deliberately asking questions and not getting anything like it when I tried to meditate.

"You're not relaxed about it." She consulted the darkened panel. "Obviously you relax interrogating professionally and not in 'trying' to meditate. You should just drift into it easily."

With my eyes lightly closed, I went down into my presumed Alpha levels. I took each step, visualizing the rainbow and my passive scene. I walked down a dozen steps into my Workshop, which I mentally equipped with various articles of furniture. I even put in a couple of imaginary assistants, feeling I might need them at this point. And, then, I imagined a large Screen in a luminous white frame. Eyes still shut, I visualized the panel of lights in the center of the Screen, all brightly Red.

As if at a distance, I heard Dawn's voice.

"The lights are all on and they're staying on."

I opened my eyes. The lights stayed lit for a few moments, then quickly fell away.

Dawn seemed strangely impressed. "It's really exciting to see all that Alpha at once."

I laid it all to my Alpha-training. "Perhaps there is some validity to all that mind-schooling."

I decided I would try looking into the body of somebody I didn't even know, just opening my mind to anyone who needed help.

Dawn allowed me to roam at will through the mysterious maze of the subconscious, watching silently as I made this curious journey into the unknown.

Again I dropped down into my levels, quickly getting into my Workshop and thrusting my unformed subject on the silver Screen. There was not even the outline of a human form, just a vague, yet insistent, presence. As I had in class, I imagined myself inside a body. It was not until my mind's eye had by stages reached the abdominal area that I saw a dark alarming mass and quickly brought my exploration to a halt. It had been a very disconcerting experience.

A flood of red lights had marked my fantasy.

I saw Dawn checking the Biofeedback record with a frown.

"Very curious," she said. "Were you blocking something?"

I stared for a moment. "Why do you say that?"

She picked up a section of the tape which mirrored the uneven course of my brainwaves. "Instead of the usual vertical slanting lines, there's a leveling out here, with a horizontal break."

I nodded slowly. "I found something very disagreeable."

It was a rather eerie feeling. I didn't have the name of the person, and the face on my imaginary Screen was just a blurred outline, but the abdominal mass seemed very real, and it seemed to me that in the ether somewhere I was picking out a message sent on a rather feeble transmitter.

Still visualizing, I made continuing efforts to re-create the face, as I had the feeling of somebody in sad straits, but nothing came of it. And I was left with a feeling of hopelessness, mine or another's.

I cleared my throat to speak, and felt a rasp of pain.

"I have had a dry, scratchy throat," I said, "ever since I lectured around the country, in Tampa, Florida, one day and Seattle the next."

"Why not take a subjective approach?"

I regarded her doubtfully. "What does that mean?"

"You could visualize your vocal chords, perhaps, in a relaxed sort of way, and see if it will ease the strain."

It seemed worth a try. My trouble may very well have

been psychosomatic by now. A subconscious expression of protest against any future tours that would take me from home. Or it could have been psychosomatic in the first place; I suddenly recalled using my ailing throat to justify cutting the trip short.

She repeated her suggestion. "Visualize or meditate in any way that will invoke Alpha and relax your throat."

Immediately I closed my eyes, gradually relaxing each muscle of the body, as suggested by Alexander. This took a minute or two, and then I went into my levels. I visualized myself on the Screen of my Mind, selecting my likeness from the jacket of the book I had discussed on the recent tour.

I examined the interior of my throat, but instead of seeing it as red and dry, I deliberately pictured it as mildly pink and moist. The vocal chords were warm and soft to the touch, rested and relaxed, fully restored, ready to speak out resonantly and painlessly.

I opened my eyes. The panel was lit up like a Christmas tree.

Dawn had a pleased look.

"Whatever you're doing is producing a shower of Alpha."

As before, the lights flickered out. The second session had ended. I had a late lunch, and then started home, hoping to beat the traffic. Instead I ran smack into it. But instead of fretting and fuming, I listened to the car radio, enjoying the music, listened to the news, without enjoying that, and finally, very much relaxed, drew up to my house two hours later. I read awhile, watched television, meditated some, on myself and another, then decided to retire. I brushed my teeth and made a singular discovery. As I opened my mouth, there was no pain, and no visible redness.

In the morning, I yawned tentatively. There was no rasping dryness or scratchiness. After six weeks, my sore throat finally seemed to have left me. One way or another, I had programmed myself to health.

Chapter 14

The Dagger of the Mind

Dawn was not surprised at my news. "Relax and get well," she said. She was inclined to be talkative, as if trying to draw me out.

As I mentioned that I still seemed to be blocking out the abdominal mass, she looked down at the tape and laughed more in wonder than amusement. "At the word *block*, the vertical line flattened out, just as it did before."

"What does that mean?"

"That you're being honest, you're blocking even as you use the word."

I had gone back to performing for the panel. "I think I'll meditate and see if I can get anything more on my unknown."

She laughed again. "At the use of the word *meditate*, there were instant waves of Alpha."

Just the thought of the two words—*block* and *meditate*—was enough to elicit the electronic response associated with each concept.

I began to concentrate. Was it possible to tune into somebody so obviously intangible? I had seen psychics pick up on people they had no conscious knowledge of and describe them perfectly, but generally they tuned in through somebody who knew the subject. I really had little to go on, except for that feeling of despair I had associated with the forbidding mass.

Dawn seemed sympathetic, but it was clearly outside her province, except for what it did for my Alpha.

"Think of whatever you like," she said.

"I surprised myself once by tuning into a ten-year-old

boy with a visual problem, and again, somebody's mother in the hospital, so maybe it will happen again."

She smiled noncommittally.

I dropped down into my imaginary Workshop once more and put a body with a dark abdominal mass on my Screen. I made no effort to pick out a face, but allowed my mind to drift lazily down the hazy outline of a human form. I got the impression that the figure was male and middle-aged, fifty-five years old, and then, keeping my eyes closed, I tried to visualize the face belonging to this body. It was to no avail, and I found myself shaking my head disconsolately.

I had not specifically told Dawn what I was doing, but I could hear her say, "You must be blocking again; the line just flattened out."

I opened my eyes. Every button on the panel was dark. My Alpha was conspicuous by its absence.

Gently Dawn made an effort to draw me off from my visual impasse by resorting to a type of questioning which had previously brought on an Alpha state.

Still monitoring her machine closely, she began to explore my own philosophical content. What, for instance, did I think of Freud and his concept of the sex drive being paramount? Or was the primary human motivation the equally primitive desire for survival?

I found myself replying that it was neither of these.

"What do you think it is?" she asked.

"A desire for social approval."

She seemed unimpressed.

"Actually," I said, "motivation varies with man's development and his sense of purpose. In adolescence a surging sexual instinct makes this appear the dominant drive. But it still relates to a desire for approval, by the girl, his peers, himself. In his twenties, thirties and forties, he is caught up in a struggle for money and influence, keyed to recognition and approval. As he passes into his fifties, with the waning of his sexual powers, sex seems to assume precedence once again, but actually he is more fearful of a loss of approval than of sex, since the flame of desire is no longer there."

I looked up to see the board lit up, and Dawn smiling encouragingly. "That makes sense," she said.

"You must remember that Freud, like so many people, saw life out of a narrow frame of reference. He was of bourgeois Viennese Jewish stock, passionately devoted to his mother; and because of his inhibitions, he was inclined to overdramatize the business of sex."

My thinking had set off a cascade of lights—a statement of truth if the subconscious was to be believed.

The little man had as much opportunity for self-approval as the captain of industry. I recalled the old Italian shoeshine man I had once interviewed on the Staten Island ferry. He was never happy unless his customer's satisfied smile was reflected in the shiny tops of his shoes. What a fortunate man!

As *The Prophet* sayeth: "Work is love made visible."

My mind drifted off into the hazy fugue of meditation, and I saw an attractive young woman shattered by a recent love affair. I saw her face clearly now on my Screen, through the misty framework of my mind. She was weeping, and her dark eyes were mirrored with despair.

What could I tell her as I considered her anxious face, except that she was far too young and pretty to let any man destroy her life? She had become fat, and the buoyancy had gone out of her voice and manner.

I had seen her only the day before. "It is me that bothers me," she had said. "Why did I make such a fool of myself? He had me changing my hair style, my clothes, the way I talked. He even made me promise I would quit my job and stay home."

He had swept her off her feet. "It was the fantasy every girl dreams of. He was Prince Charming. He brought flowers and candy. And he wrote poetry. It was all moonlight and roses."

I kept my eyes closed and hoped for an Alpha-like burst of wisdom that would enable me to comfort her.

On my Screen, she was still sobbing. "He made me over, and I was no longer me. I didn't know who I was. It was all so confusing."

That was it, of course. She had gotten away from her own center. One thought tumbled out after the other until I felt I could reconstruct the events that had led to her demoralization. She had made the mistake of surrendering her values, and was left with no hard core of her own to fall back on when the break came.

I sighed and found myself staring into a panel of lights.

The third session was over, but I had my stop to make in Hollywood. The girl was waiting for me anxiously. I looked at her unhappy face. "Dry your tears," I said, "and listen." I proceeded to unfold what had come to me in meditation, and found her nodding.

"Exactly," she said with a throb of anger. "He tried to take me over."

"But you let him, so it was your doing."

She frowned, knitting her eyebrows into an even line.

"One day he told me he didn't like the way I dressed, and I told him I was through."

"That should have helped; you were back on center, your ego intact."

"But a week later he called and was Prince Charming again." She gulped. "We started living together, and I thought everything was fine. And then he wandered off, without a word. I called him frantically, but he wouldn't come to the phone."

"Did you finally reach him?"

I thought the poor girl was about to break into tears all over again. "He told me he never wanted to see me again."

I closed my eyes and pictured him in my Workshop.

"I suppose he went back to his mother."

She looked up, gaping.

"How did you know about his mother?"

"He is thirty-five years old?"

Her jaw dropped. "I never mentioned his age."

"You never had a chance," I said. "His mother will always have first claim. He is troubled by his own sexuality, and the moment it looked like wedding bells he ran for cover." I saw it all on my Screen, and I was no more psychic than the average.

She appeared to be going over the relationship. "All right," she said. "I accept what you have said. But why so cruel?"

"Because of a dominating mother, he had to feel superior to somebody. So he came back to you."

"So that he could have the satisfaction of dropping

me?" Her eyes flashed. "Why, that creep," she said with her old sparkle. "I'm glad to be rid of him."

I kept thinking uneasily of the dark mass. At first, I thought it might relate to somebody I knew, but the feeling was growing that it was just somebody out there into whose frequency I had somehow tuned in, leaving my subconscious open.

I had the feeling his hour was drawing close. It was depressing, and seemed to serve no purpose. For I was obviously neither a healer nor a doctor, and sickness made me uneasy. I tried just concentrating on the lights and made another discovery. When I said or thought anything that expressed Alpha, the lights lit up, regardless of the voltage demand. Dawn had increased the voltage from five to ten microvolts, requiring that much more electrical energy on my part. At first, as I tried to think them on, the buttons remained in darkness. But when I mentioned that I would meditate, as before, on the rolling sea, there was a flurry of lights and I heard a strange rasping noise.

I caught a look of surprise on Dawn's face. "You put out so much Alpha then," she said, "that the needle scratched across the EEG tape."

Obviously an electrical potential opened up all sorts of interesting possibilities. I could see myself lighting a room as I entered, moving the remote-controlled garage door, even powering an elevator.

I allowed my mind to wander with my eyes open. The black blob, unpredictably, loomed large in my mind, and I tried putting it on my imaginary Screen. It kept fading.

"I'm still blocking," I said, and immediately drew a response from Dawn. "There's that line flattening out again."

A whole new concept of communication was beginning to manifest itself.

"The articulation of mere words, such as *meditation* or *blocking*," I said, "obviously has no special sonar action on either the lights or the tape. They are plainly symbols of the thought wave which produced them. So merely by expressing thought waves, one should be able to communicate directly with another human being as long as the symbols have the same significance for both."

Dawn was not about to commit herself, but she was

open and interested, with the earmark of a true scientist, an insatiable curiosity. "There's no point to closing off possibilities until they have been investigated. But we have not yet advanced to where we can fully explore all these areas and accept or reject them."

"And we won't," I said, "until researchers have been trained to produce Alpha and Theta at will, materializing subjective experiences they can check out."

"Unfortunately," she said, "much of the laboratory research is being done by people in Beta who have never experimented themselves with producing Alpha or Theta waves."

It seemed incredible that anybody could reach for the clouds while sitting blindfolded in the small prison of his mind. They seemed to have completely overlooked the bold, boundless spirit which had raised man out of the animal kingdom and made the universe his backyard.

Without saying a word, I had lit up the panel and made it stay lit.

Words were not the only daggers of the mind.

Chapter 15

Hypnosis

"What is the difference," I said, "between hypnosis and what we are trying to do in Alpha?"

Dawn's answer came as a surprise. "Nothing, as far as I can see."

"Ours seems a sort of auto-hypnosis," I conceded.

"There is nothing wrong with hypnosis as long as it is constructively used," she said. "It has just been misunderstood over the years."

"How about girls who claim they have been seduced by hypnotists?" I asked, thinking of a very specific case.

"You're always hearing that," she replied, "but nobody can be made to do something contrary to his nature."

"The hypnotist may be bringing out a part of their nature better left unexplored."

"In the last analysis," she said, "you do it yourself. The suggestion is planted in the subconscious mind, and the individual does the rest. People who take Alpha courses, or submit to Biofeedback, generally want to do something about themselves, and so usually have an impressionable subconscious."

I thought back a few years to another project. "I can remember a case where a man had hypnotized his subject in her sleep and influenced her behavior."

She nodded. "Why not? The individual is in either Alpha or Theta, or a mixture of the two, in sleep, and so extremely susceptible to suggestion."

She had hypnotized her own ten-year-old daughter in her sleep to improve her daily habits. "She had been leaving her room untidy, and so I suggested that she clean after herself every day. This worked for a few days, and

170

then her interest flagged, so I repeated the suggestion, this time specifying that she would get pleasure out of cleaning her room. This made it fun, and provided a positive motivation."

Her daughter had been lackadaisical about her schoolwork, and Dawn had similarly suggested that she apply herself industriously both in the classroom and in her homework, enjoying her new productivity. And this, too, had worked, just as it had for Stew Esposito's toilet-trained son.

It also reminded me of Lennie Weitz sleeping through his class and winding up, nevertheless, as the star pupil.

How did the subject, his five senses turned off in sleep, respond to a suggestion that he had not consciously heard? Obviously there was transference of thought, in terms of familiar word symbols, picked up in subconscious communication.

"There's nothing weird or esoteric about hypnosis," Dawn observed. "Everybody is hypnotized every day of his life, over the radio and television, in the newspapers and magazines, in daily conversation with friends, relatives, and by such authority figures as doctors, lawyers, teachers, public officials. We are constantly bombarded with suggestions to buy this or that, do this or that, go here or there. And quite often it works, or the suggestions, particularly the commercial variety, wouldn't be continued."

Only the night before, at ten-minute intervals, a television voice had kept insisting this was the flu season, and that as we came down with flu we should try his marvelous product. It would get rid of all the symptoms, he promised as he pantomimed all the miseries of the flu. I turned him off before my throat started scratching again.

"The Alpha mind," said Dawn, "would automatically tune out most of this garbage, conserving time and energy for some useful activity."

"In other words, I might hear the soft music as I worked at my typewriter but would tune out the commercial."

"If your Alpha mind had decided that the commercial was distracting to your creative process."

In this very awareness lay the individual's defense.

Playing tennis, I had fallen and torn several ligaments in my right arm, and shattered the synovial capsule containing the elbow fluid. It had been an excruciating experience, and six weeks later the motion of the arm was still painfully restricted. I could not bring my right hand to my mouth or head and was compelled to eat, brush my teeth, and comb my hair with my left hand. At the urging of physican friends, I went to a prominent orthopedic surgeon. He scanned the X-rays, took my arm out of its sling, and moved it tentatively, as far as it would go.

He gave me a solemn look. "I can't guarantee," he said, "that you will regain full use of your arm."

I returned his gaze evenly, and spoke slowly, in measured tones. "I have no doubt that my arm will regain its full strength and that full motion will be restored."

"Fine," he said with a smile, and I could tell from the distant look in his eyes that his mind was already on his next appointment.

As a doctor's wife, Dawn had been listening with special interest.

I moved my right arm in every direction for her benefit. "That was six weeks ago," I said, "and today my arm is as good as new."

"Did you go into physiotherapy?" she asked.

"I had two sessions," I said, "and I did a few minutes of isometric exercises at home every day, constantly visualizing the arm as being well and totally functional. I felt he had laid a negative thought on me, and I knew I had to counter it somehow, or the image of a restricted arm could persist and perhaps prevail."

The experience had provided an earlier example of positive visualization. I had fallen on my inside elbow with the full weight of my body, and the elbow had crunched out of joint, leaving my arm dangling by the skin. As my companions helped me off the court, I placed my left hand on the elbow and saw it in place. That instant, the elbow slid into the joint.

Edward Robinson, a Buffalo attorney and judge, drove me seventeen miles over a bumpy road to a Buffalo hospital.

There, a doctor surveyed the X-rays, announced there were no broken bones, and said I had contusions.

"Contusions!" exclaimed Judge Robinson. "The man dislocated his arm."

The doctor fingered my arm. "I see no dislocation."

"He put it back in place himself."

The doctor gave him a patronizing smile. "Nobody can put his own elbow back in place."

Ed Robinson exploded. "I'm a judge," he said, "and when I say he put his arm in place, he put his arm in place."

In keeping with my Alpha-training, I had a feeling of fusion with sundry people and events at scattered places. I would think of certain people and would express the thought that they contact me. In a few days, I heard by mail from Bill Schwartz of the Meditation Institute in Milwaukee, and he advised that the information I wanted was on its way. I wondered about psychic Maya Perez's whereabouts, and a letter promptly arrived from Maya Perez, giving her address in Balboa, California, and her telephone number.

Involuntarily I kept seeing the black abdominal mass, with its connotation of cancer in the lower chest or stomach area. I had a foreboding of death, but at the same time realized that the victim was neither a friend nor relative, but still somebody whose name would be familiar. As the image grew darker in my mind, I felt death more imminent. I consulted the obituary pages. The impression of death was so strong I felt somebody was trying to tell me something. The night after I scanned the obituaries, I was lying sleepless and heard a radio voice mention that a best-selling author had just died. I sat up, but the voice had moved on.

In the morning, I went through the newspapers and found a half column devoted to the writer's death. He had died in his fifty-fifth year, of cancer. I felt a twinge of regret, feeling there had been a message for me had I the wit to perceive it.

I mentioned my frustrating experience to mind-trainer Pat Patrick.

"Could I have done anything?" I asked.

She thought a moment. "From the inner contact that had been established, you could have sent out thoughts of help to this individual."

"But I wasn't sure of the individual."

"How else," she said, "would this appeal have reached you?"

"I didn't want to appear foolish."

"It wouldn't have been foolish to release a kind, loving, healing thought, wherever it went." She smiled. "Even if it only came back to you."

Dawn had shown no interest in my visualization of the cancerous mass, presumably considering it highly apocryphal, and negative at that. But now she regarded me curiously.

"Does that image still keep recurring?"

I shook my head. "No, it seemed to stop with a man's death."

She looked down quickly at the rasp of the EEG tape.

"Well," she said, "you're no longer blocking. All the lines are nicely slanted, and you are in a very fine Alpha form." Death had obviously removed any tenuous connection I had with him.

What was there about visualization and meditation that seemed so much more effective than concentrating on a desired goal with the purely objective mind?

"What is the difference between positive thinking and what we are doing?"

Dawn looked at me without replying, as if wanting me to think it out for myself.

"Even if it's positive thinking, I suppose, it's still Beta, and so limited by the Beta mind."

She nodded encouragingly, shifting her glance to see how many lights I had lit.

"In Alpha, on the other hand, you would relax, seeing the situation in its full context, not only as it affected you, but associates, friends, relatives, the community."

She seemed more concerned about what the lights were doing than what I was saying. A few lights quickly flickered on and off, and that was all.

I rummaged around in my mind. "True positive thinking is a consequence of an altered consciousness, not its cause," I said finally.

Dawn's eyes brightened, and so did the panel. All eight lights flashed on at once, and stayed on for several seconds.

"What we may be establishing here," I said, "is that the mind in its totality is a master computer. When it grinds and churns and comes up with the right answer, the lights go on because Alpha has the answers when Beta has trouble phrasing the questions."

The goals were similar in positive thinking and Alpha programming—success and happiness. But limited Beta couldn't distinguish happiness from success. They could be vastly different. I recalled two youthful writers who had achieved overnight fame through persevering. They had thought positively, and it had helped them succeed beyond their fondest hopes.

And then with the world's adulation in their grasp, each had killed himself.

I had puzzled over these suicides. The two men had not only achieved their apparent goals but had gained a success that the most gifted vainly strove to achieve. Now, putting the puzzle on the Screen of the Mind, I felt I understood what had happened. Feeling a depressing sense of emptiness and unfulfillment, they had anticipated a marvelous transformation with success, and when they still felt empty and unrealized, they were overwhelmed. They had no other mountains to climb.

Had they established contact with their inner being, they might have known where to look for what they were lacking. It was in the universe around them, and it was part of themselves. But, sadly, they didn't even know what was missing.

"It all begins with the individual," Dawn observed. "All we can do is give him the tools to explore his oneness with the oneness around him."

"And to know his own needs?"

"That's part of it."

"And how to fulfill them."

"Exactly."

My experience with Biofeedback was doubly revealing. I could produce Alpha by simulating Alpha-like sensations experienced during my classroom training, and I could produce Alpha by reproducing those thoughts, images, or sensations that had turned on the lights.

"So now that I can produce Alpha at will, what do we do with it?"

Dawn smiled. "What would you like to do with it?"

For most of my life, I had been plagued by insomnia. "I must have had a very frightening childhood," I said. "I keep getting up in the night and can't get back to sleep."

"Did you have falling dreams as a child?"

"I didn't know there were any other kind."

"I would have thought," she said, "that your Yoga-training would have helped you."

"It did help me get to sleep. I was able to nap during the day for the first time, just lying down and relaxing without trying to sleep."

"Why not try that at night?"

"It only works when I'm physically weary. But after sleeping two or three hours, I'm usually wide awake."

"Try getting down to Theta. That's four to seven brainwaves per second, as you know, and is normally marked by drowsiness."

"And how will I do that?"

"You're probably already producing Theta, along with the Alpha. It's just a matter of setting a machine, slowing down the brainwaves to a visual pattern producing Theta. That's obviously the value of Biofeedback."

"But I don't have a machine in my bedroom."

"No, but knowing what mentally puts you in Theta, you can then recall it. The slower rhythm obviously encourages sleep."

"Will I program myself as I'm retiring, or after I've awakened?"

She laughed uproariously.

"Here you are, speaking of sleeping in one breath and in the next programming yourself to wake up."

"How is that?"

"You speak of getting up in the night as if it's a foregone conclusion, just as that surgeon spoke of your arm. You saw it when he did it, but not when you do it."

"I had the problem before the thought."

"Whatever the original problem, it's a new problem now. You have given your subconscious a wake-up alert for so long that it's now second nature. We'll just have to reprogram you completely. To avoid conflict, stop thinking that your sleep will be interrupted. Banish that thought completely."

I couldn't help but smile. "Would you call that positive thinking?"

"Right. But it won't do the job itself; it just helps create the proper climate."

Chapter 16

Under the Influence

Dawn's suggestion seemed to do it.

I felt unusually fresh and alert from two relatively good nights. I had awakened once or twice, then quickly gone back to sleep. Normally I would have read a book, watched the Late Show, or even worked awhile.

The long drive to Pasadena, usually tedious, seemed almost pleasant, as my new energy gave me an easy command of the road.

I observed not only the passing cars but the passengers, and occasionally smiled at a pretty motorist. I wondered why I had ever thought the trip a chore.

I arrived in record time and parked my car with a smile, thinking what I would do to the Alpha lights.

I was still smiling as Dawn rigged the electrodes to my head.

"You must be sleeping well," she said. "You don't look as grainy as usual."

"I've slept like a log, waking up briefly, then slipping right back to sleep."

"You obviously eliminated the negative thought that you'd wake up and not get back to sleep."

"I also did some positive visualization."

"Oh?" said Dawn, fumbling with the attachments.

"I pictured myself watching a television game show, and my eyes got so heavy I couldn't keep them open."

"Were you in bed?"

"No, on a chaise longue, but it works in bed, too."

She had finished with the electrodes and turned to the panel.

My mind was unusually restless. I kept thinking of publishers, agents, attorneys, slick tradespeople and how I wished I were a mechanic or electrician. I wandered on to the morning news—inflation, recession, violence, conflict in the Mideast, the apparent inevitability of mass killing in an absurd world.

Not one light blinked on. I kept staring at the panel, and still not a single light.

"Is it hooked up?"

Dawn examined the various connections. "I don't understand. It's the first time you haven't gone right into Alpha."

I tried visualization, but not even this brought the customary response. "Why doesn't the thing light up?"

"Are you repeating what you did to light it up before?"

"I've gone through the whole routine, meditating, going into my levels, but"—I hesitated—"it's not quite the same."

She leaped in eagerly. "In what way?"

"I'm trying too hard, like a baseball pitcher aiming a ball instead of throwing it naturally."

It reminded me of my first session with Alexander, when I briefly despaired of closing off my conscious mind.

"I have no idea why I can't slide into Alpha, with all the practice I've had."

"Perhaps," she said, "it has something to do with your being fresh and alert."

I groaned. "Do I have to be tired to be in Alpha?"

Obviously other people were going into Alpha while they were comfortably rested, so my reaction presumably had something to do with my peculiar thinking patterns.

I felt frustrated, staring at the darkened panel. "Maybe I should call it a day and come back when I'm tired."

Dawn was more persevering. "Why not relax into the techniques you learned?"

I methodically went into my levels, closing my eyes and allowing the colors of the rainbow to merge successively into each other; I counted down slowly from twenty-one, visualizing a stone step for each number, then imagined a large Workshop with walnut paneling, which I began to furnish elaborately, with overstuffed couches and chairs, a color television set, a large worktable, a typewriter with a magic touch.

I installed a large Screen in this Workshop, and now placed a familiar face on this Screen. My own. I saw myself as first a boy, then a young man, and now in my middle years. Happily, my features remained the same, free of lines and wrinkles, and I thought of myself as ever youthful, constantly rejuvenated by Yoga and a mind that refused to accept the popular notion of dying.

My thoughts drifted naturally to the national obsession with age. I had declined to give my age to a newspaperwoman, with the jest that I was ageless.

"Why," the unamused lady reporter had asked, "can't you simply give your age without making a deal out of it?"

Had she asked, I would have shared the thoughts now passing through my mind. I would have told her that once a maturing person thinks himself a particular age, whether fifty, fifty-five, sixty, then he begins to age in that pattern. He begins to cut down on exercise, and to close off options, to conform to the stereotype for his age. Soon he is thinking more of retiring than living and is the age he says and more. Comedian Jack Benny's joke about being thirty-nine was more than a pleasantry and had something to do with his staying youthful at eighty. He had programmed himself.

I found Dawn eyeing me curiously. "Whatever you were thinking sure turned on the Alpha."

In deliberately dropping into my levels, I had apparently slipped out of my Beta world for the time.

"I was thinking how people allow themselves to be brainwashed into senility."

"Yes?"

"Looking at a man of fifty, I often see a fading, defeated, frustrated figure, already thinking in terms of the scrap pile. Now if I associate myself with that age, the first thing I know, I'm like that man."

Dawn had the happy facility of instant comprehension. "And you'll begin to age like him?"

"Exactly, for the mind, as we are finding out, can help us thrust our way to infinity or, turned inward, gradually destroy us."

"In other words, if you keep saying you're fifty or sixty, you'll perform accordingly."

"Since we commonly associate the latter age with retirement, you would have to be thinking in terms of your pension and some Valhalla by the sea, where you can play shuffleboard, darts, and bridge while waiting for the undertaker."

"And what do you suggest?"

"Be your own person, think ageless, and stay away from the doctors."

I found Dawn laughing quietly to herself. "That really touched off the lights."

My Alpha interlude over, my Beta mind strained for information about the patients under Biofeedback therapy.

I considered first the case of the man who had lost use of his right arm in an automobile accident. He had been unable to move a muscle when he first began visualizing in Alpha, then gradually moved to the EMG, the electromyograph, which tested his muscle response to his own brainwaves.

"He is doing very well," Dawn reported. "He is able to clench his fingers when he couldn't even move them before."

It had taken six weeks of Alpha-training before he was ready for the electromyograph.

"It was a job," said Dawn, "convincing him that visualization could help his arm."

"Does he have trouble visualizing his muscles moving?"

"The EEG lights up whenever he repeats mentally the visual picture that lit it up the first time."

"That was when he visualized a helpful hand moving the muscle of his arm?"

"We vary the image from time to time, keeping the idea of help from outside. Variety keeps the patient from getting bored."

Some patients had responded especially well to the visualization treatment for migraine headaches. And anybody troubled by this agonizing problem could easily appreciate what a boon this could be.

I had picked up a report of the National Migraine Foundation. "Were you aware," I said, "that ninety percent of the headaches treated by physicians are psychogenic in origin?"

She moved her shoulders slightly. "I feel ninety percent of all illness is largely psychogenic."

"Eight percent is circulatory in nature, and only two percent organic in origin."

"You're no healthier than your circulatory system, but the mind influences even that."

I read on: " 'Some eighty percent of the migraine sufferers are women, hard-driving, keen intellectually, compulsive workers.' " I paused and looked over at her. "What will Women's Lib say about that?"

"Women," she commented, "may be more sensitive, and are certainly more emotional, than men."

"Then would you say it was a tension syndrome?"

"I have never known a migraine sufferer who also didn't suffer from tension."

"So deep inner relaxation, brought on by Alpha-thinking, might be a specific solution?"

"It certainly would be helpful."

Without being deeply relaxed, there was little chance of a subject increasing the blood flow to his hand, as the patient with Raynaud's Phenomenon had done with visualization and concentration.

"Obviously," said Dawn, "the secondary effect on the cranial circulation would not have occurred without mind control and relaxation."

There were plainly many thoughts that would bring blood to the fingers.

"Suppose they visualized warming their hands over a hot stove?"

"That might suggest more heat than warmth."

"Would sexual fantasies produce the desired warmth?"

She laughed. "If they gave a person a warm feeling inside, yes."

The session ended without my discovering why I should not be at a creative peak when feeling my best physically. Nevertheless, my psychic awareness appeared to be developing. I would now frequently anticipate a name before it was mentioned to me. A Malibu realtor, Alex Reachi, groped for the family name of a wealthy woman whose husband had purchased property nearby.

"I just can't think of it," he said.

"Is it Guinness?" I ventured.

I heard his gasp on the telephone. "How did you know?"

"I was just guessing." And I was, in a way.

I had been sleeping progressively better, until one evening at dinner, I had my first coffee in months. I stirred sleeplessly all night, and in the morning was so bedraggled that I had to resist an impulse to cancel my session.

When I finally arrived, I was grateful for the opportunity to sit down and relax. I allowed my mind to drift idly, too fatigued to concentrate on any single thought very long.

I barely heard Dawn say in a puzzled tone, "That's odd; you're turning on the Alpha lights while you're complaining about being tired."

I opened my eyes, and sure enough, the panel was lit up. "Maybe it's not-thinking that does it."

Her eyes bright with excitement, Dawn questioned me about my work habits.

"I usually write at night, in the quiet preceding midnight, and sometimes afterward."

"You must be weary after a long day."

"I suppose so, but that's when it seems to come easier."

"You work also in the morning?"

"I usually edit what I did the night before, but this is routine."

"It would seem to me," she said, "that tired, you are more prone to Alpha because you are resting the sensory Beta mind, and so permitting Alpha to come through more readily."

"You mean the more mentally fatigued I am the clearer my thinking?"

"As far as your creative capacity goes. In the morning, for instance, when relatively fresh, you are doing the rational work of Beta, sharpening and rearranging your work, approaching it almost as if it were somebody else's."

"That's true, but it seems to me that the fresher I am, the more aware I should be of what's going on around me."

"Right, but only with the five senses reflected by Beta."

It was an idea I was not ready to accept, for I knew my newspaper work in the past had often suffered from my being fatigued.

"But don't you see," she said eagerly, "journalism is a Beta function, reporting what you observe, seldom scratching below the surface of events?"

I considered for a moment, then made a truly self-willed Taurean observation. "I still don't see why I should be thinking better when my mind doesn't seem to be turning over."

Suddenly, out of the past, I recalled Charles Edison telling me that his father, Thomas Edison, had conceived his inventions in the drowsy state preceding his little catnaps. He had certainly not been fresh and alert at the time, and it would have been interesting to see what he would have done with the electroencephalograph attached to his head. Probably invented a better one.

The body took weeks, months, to overcome assaults mounted by its own mind. But in a week, a day, an hour, perhaps a second, the mind could be turned around and begin to correct whatever damage it had done its shell.

But to achieve the relaxation necessary for healing, it was obviously essential to stabilize Alpha-Theta thinking to the point where it could be held at will, not flashing on and off like a traffic blinker.

Unless I could light up the Alpha panel and keep it lit for an extended period, I had manifestly not gained true mastery over my brain and body.

Floating my mind, I cocked a quizzical eye at the darkened panel and drew a deep breath, deliberately inducing a tingling sensation in the pit of my stomach.

The lights went on, and as I continued to regard the panel in a contemplative fashion, they stayed on. There was not a wink, a blink, or a nod. I stared at the lights, and they stared back, all eight of them.

"Whatever are you doing?" said Dawn. "I've never seen them remain on so long."

"Maybe the machine is stuck."

I kept my eye on the panel.

She consulted her watch. "You've kept the Alpha on for more than a minute."

My attention wandered, and the lights suddenly blinked off.

"One minute and fifteen seconds," she said exultantly.

"Is that a world's record?"

She bobbed her head, marveling. "It is for my experience, both here and during my research stint at the Veterans Hospital in Los Angeles."

I tried reconstructing my feelings.

"I hypnotized the lights."

She laughed. "You what?"

"I decided that unless I could keep them on I wasn't making progress."

She checked the myograph, attached to my right elbow. "The needle shows that your muscle is responding normally."

She gave me an uncertain smile. "You're not serious about hypnotizing the machine?"

"Actually I told myself I could keep the lights on as long as I kept staring at the panel a certain way."

"But what were you thinking?"

"I kept thinking of the panel all lit up."

"But you have done that before."

"Not with the same confidence and motivation."

She frowned. "The confidence comes from having done it before, but what new motivation . . . ?" Her voice trailed off.

"I couldn't let that panel get the better of me."

She looked concerned. "Are you feeling tired?"

"I never felt better."

"But you seem to do better fatigued."

It was incongruous that I should not do my best when I felt my best. And since I was convinced that Alpha-thinking was superior to Beta, I was interested in synchronizing my peak energy level with the Alpha meditative process.

"Thinking it over, I felt I was not getting the maximum result."

Dawn waited for me to go on.

"My sluggish mind was naturally reflecting the slower rhythms of Alpha and some Theta. But while my creative faculty may have been on the increase, I was not always energetic enough to take advantage of it."

"In other words, you wanted to be creative and energetic at the same time?"

"Isn't that what we're trying to do?"

"Precisely." She had allowed me to figure it out for myself.

Actually Alpha output stemmed from a combination of factors, not the least of which, I suspected, was the detached way I found myself looking at the lights, and the deep rhythmical breathing, both relaxing and mind-expanding at the same time.

To be scientific or mechanistic—one had to repeat a phenomenon. So I took a deep Yogic breath, right down to the diaphragm, inhaling and exhaling slowly; then with the same hazy detachment invoking the same tingling sensation, I again eyed the Alpha panel. As before, all the lights came on, and stayed on. The thought came to mind that if I moved my head the lights would vanish. In response, one light flickered out. I banished the thought and concentrated on keeping the lights on. I felt my mind drifting easily, even while I was aware of what I was trying to do. An eternity seemed to pass, but I knew it was only seconds. The conscious and the unconscious mind—the subconscious—appeared to be merging, as Elmer Green had suggested they might with practice. My stomach kept tingling, and I tried keeping the sensation alive. I knew it had something to do with keeping the lights on.

Finally, in this curious dichotomy, the conscious part of me grew tired of the game and I averted my gaze. The charm was broken, the panel went blank. But I had kept the lights on for almost two minutes.

Dawn was visibly impressed. "You have apparently learned to control your Alpha mind and to relax at will."

There was no overnight transformation, but I did feel an altered awareness, which brought its changes almost imperceptibly. I felt calmer, more assured, less irascible, even patient. Even so, I would not have given these changes another thought had it not been for marveling friends. They kept telling me I was more mellow, and pleasant, better company, until I wondered what sort of ogre I had been before. I had stopped reacting to the disappointments I would have once carried to sleep with me. I delayed decisions, giving myself time to meditate, and discovered very often that no action was necessary. The situation resolved itself.

My insomnia was at the vanishing point. I fell asleep watching television, and if I woke during the night, all I had to imagine was that I was watching the same show that put me to sleep. I even found myself sleeping through until morning. If it had not been television, I would have improvised something else. What worked for some didn't for others. But once anybody became susceptible to self-suggestion in Alpha, I was sure any visualization inducing drowsiness would serve the purpose.

There was no one special way, even in stopping smoking. Even a negative suggestion could be effective. "Visualize your lungs as black and sooty from years of smoking, then with each puff of a cigarette see the film of soot becoming thicker, spreading to the bronchial tubes and the larynx." That had worked for many chain-smokers. On the positive side, the lungs could be visualized as pink and healthy and perfect, the way you wanted them to be. But since most people with bad habits were negatively oriented, the first suggestion seemed to offer a better prospect.

"Unfortunately," agreed Dawn, "that's the kind of world we live in."

Chapter 17

The Prize Pupil

Dr. Balog's cases were already recovered or improved, for the most part, and I had no way, aside from testimonials, of observing their progress from the beginning. I looked around for a test case of my own and came up with sixteen-year-old Greg Porter, a schoolboy tennis player, whose tennis had been interrupted by traumatic arthritis of the right arm. Young Greg had consulted three of the most respected orthopedic specialists in Southern California. He was told the condition was irreversible and his arm would always be restricted.

He was by no means a basket case; he could play basketball, but he couldn't reach or extend himself, stretch high to serve, dunk a basket, or spike a volleyball. For an athletically inclined boy, it was a disaster.

Greg seemed an ideal subject. He could have passed for the All-American teen-ager on the verge of manhood. He was tall and lanky, well over six feet, with blond good looks, wavy hair, and dreamy blue eyes. He was ideally built for a tennis player, though he could have used a little more weight.

I explained Dr. Balog's concept of self-healing, and he nodded intelligently.

"Some people have the will to live and triumph over apparently incurable ailments. Others wish themselves into illness, often to avoid the challenges of being well."

"There's no way I don't want to get well."

The third doctor had virtually written him off.

"In time, I was told, my arm would calcify and the pain gradually go away."

I told him he would be tested for Alpha first; then

188

when he could produce Alpha at will, he would be hooked up to the EMG, the muscle-responding device, and then the thermistor, the temperature sensor.

Greg's difficulty had developed after the death of his father in a boating accident. Whether there was any psychosomatic tie-up was, of course, highly speculative. But I believed, with many men of medicine, that a good share of man's illness, if not most of it, was attributable to the mind's negative action on the body.

Greg was intrigued with the thought of just sitting in a chair, turning on lights with his mind, and healing himself. "How do I know I can produce Alpha brainwaves?"

"The younger you are, the more imagination you have, the less influenced by the rational outside world, the easier it is to produce Alpha."

Dawn immediately put him at ease. As she had with me, she attached the electrodes of the Alpha machine to his scalp and told him to visualize or think about anything that came to his mind.

"You might close your eyes," she prompted. "It usually works better that way."

Greg slumped in his chair and closed his lids.

The lights flashed on and stayed on for a few seconds.

"What voltage is he on?" I asked.

"Five microvolts for each light, for a starter, as you were."

Apparently distracted, Greg opened his eyes.

"What were you thinking?" I asked.

He smiled. "I saw myself playing tennis."

"Were you moving your elbow?"

"Oh, yes, the whole arm."

He closed his eyes, and again the panel lit up.

"He's making it look easy," I said.

"Being young has something to do with it," Dawn said, "and he's obviously creative."

"How about turning up the machine to ten volts?"

Dawn deftly adjusted the electroencephalograph.

There was no decrease in the flow of Alpha. The lights raced up and down the scale, holding for an instant before blinking off.

Suddenly the lights stayed on.

"What are you thinking now?" Dawn asked.

Without opening his eyes, Greg replied, "I just served an ace."

An ace, I explained to Dawn, was an unreturnable serve, one the opponent could not even get his racket on.

"You had to stretch high in the air and smash down on the ball," I pointed out.

His head bobbed in cheerful agreement.

Dawn looked at me questioningly. "I think," she said, "he's sufficiently in Alpha to hook up to the muscle-responder."

Greg seemed to be making unusual progress, since the man with the paralyzed arm had taken six weeks before he got this far.

Greg rubbed his eyes as the panel lit up.

"I was just playing Wimbledon," he announced matter-of-factly.

England's Wimbledon was the most prestigious of all tennis tournaments, and I wondered for a moment if Greg was putting us on.

He gave his slow, easy smile. "I was just rallying, getting the ball back, the whole thing, before I made an overhead smash."

Dawn leaned forward to attach the electrodes from the EMG, the electromyograph, to Greg's elbow. "Exactly where does it bother you?"

He pointed to the inner right elbow. "Between the two small bones."

She attached the machine just above the indicated spot, directly onto a controlling muscle.

The EEG was still connected, so Greg was now registering on two machines. Dawn stepped back and surveyed her handiwork. "We can see now how the two synchronize, mind and body."

He was still playing great tennis, visually.

"I just served another ace," he announced as all eight lights winked on and the needle on the EMG (rated from zero to forty-five microvolts) leaped forward.

The EMG was so delicate that it picked up the muscle's slightest electrical activity reflected in tiny dartings of the needle. "As long as we have movement, there is hope of normalizing the muscle," Dawn said.

"Why," I asked as the panel flashed on, "is he producing so much Alpha?"

"Younger people have more imagination, reflected in Alpha creativity, but as they get older and substitute logical thinking for the creative dreamlike state, they produce more Beta activity, and this is incorporated into their life style."

Suddenly the EMG needle flipped to the right and forty-five microvolts.

Dawn looked up in surprise. "His muscle must have jumped on that one!"

Greg opened his eyes. "It did twitch a bit."

"What were you thinking about?" she asked.

He smiled. "I just spiked a volleyball for game point."

"Volleyball?"

"Oh, yes, that's my favorite sport."

"What," I asked Dawn, "is the significance of his muscle twitching?"

"It means that he's on the road to recovery."

Even without visualization, the myograph needle had advanced to a middle position.

Dawn leaned forward. "Are you sure your arm is not throbbing?"

"Quite sure," he replied.

"Then the accelerated muscle response obviously reflects a stimulated healing process from increased blood flow."

He had closed his eyes and was now trying to visualize his arm as being completely well, the muscles smooth and hard, and the blood circulating with invigorating warmth.

His meditation was abruptly interrupted by Dawn's exclamation. "The needle is really jumping!"

It had advanced as far to the right as it could.

Dawn's face glowed with pleasure. "He's doing so well, perhaps we should try the temperature sensor the next time."

Greg's head turned slightly. "What's that?"

She explained that it would additionally stimulate the blood flow to his elbow, removing any toxic by-products of the arthritis.

"Why can't he just visualize the arthritis as disappearing?"

Dawn chuckled at my eagerness. "And exactly what would an arthritic arm look like?"

I thought for a moment. "One free of arthritis."

She shook her head. "Not substantial enough, visually."

"How about visualizing his arthritis being dissolved in warm water?"

She looked at the clock. "How about visualizing an end to a very satisfactory session?"

Greg's recovery was by no means assured. He seemed interested but not convinced, involved but not expectant. He had all the machines working for him, but it was almost a reflex action. I wondered if he would be another Biofeedback athlete.

Greg's mother was less than encouraging. "Greg," she said, "is skeptical about getting help from the Biofeedback program."

This came as no surprise.

"He has to be expectant," I said, "otherwise it may not work. Nobody gets well if he doesn't want to."

"Oh, he wants to, all right," she said. "He just doesn't see how it can happen."

That day, I saw Greg in the doctor's waiting room. "Confidence," I told him, "is half the battle."

He smiled. "All I said was that it was a unique and strange experience and I wasn't quite sure what was happening."

"In one session, you made more progress with the Alpha-testing and muscle-response machines than one man did in a dozen, and he's now moving an arm crippled in an accident."

Dawn's appearance interrupted the conversation, but only briefly. I repeated what his mother had said.

Dawn looked at Greg with concern. "You really are doing fine and should have no trouble getting back full use of your arm." As a psychologist, Dawn decided it might be time to explore the boy's attitude about his injury. "How," she asked, "did you first throw out your arm?"

"It was a carnival, a Mardi Gras at UCLA. I was trying to knock down a doll in one of these booths where you pay so much a ball and can win a prize."

"You haven't played tennis since?"

He shook his head.

"And how long ago was that?"

"Four years, about."

"But you play basketball?"

"Until my arm starts hurting."

Dawn was hooking him up to the various wires as she talked, the EEG, the EMG, and now a thermistor, registering the temperature of the left hand.

"Why the left hand," he asked, "when it's my right arm that's hurt?"

"It doesn't matter which hand, so long as you increase the blood flow."

Greg now had three machines to concentrate on, and it presented obvious difficulties. But he rose to the challenge.

The Alpha lights went on, and at the same time the needle on the EMG jumped forward.

"What," said Dawn, "were you thinking then?"

"I was just beating down John Newcombe," said Greg, speaking rather irreverently of this top tennis player.

"Was it an overhead smash?"

"All kinds of strokes," he said with his easy smile.

I had a sudden thought. "How can you play basketball and not tennis?"

"Because my elbow is involved in tennis and it hurts when I extend my arm upward or out."

There was a sound attachment to the EMG, and it now began to beep above our voices.

Dawn looked at him inquiringly.

"I saw a tennis court, and on its surface, in concrete lettering, the words, 'I will get well.' "

Dawn amended.

"I *am* getting well."

"All right, I *am* getting well."

"That's better," she said as the EMG responded.

The lids of his eyes closed.

"Are you still skeptical?"

He shook his head. "It wasn't being skeptical so much as watching and waiting."

"That's a healthy attitude," she said, "so long as you haven't closed off the possibilities."

"I wouldn't be here if I had."

The thermistor had not advanced at all.

"It's a question," explained Dawn, "of his learning to concentrate on three different machines individually and collectively; it takes some practice."

Dawn had suggested a little homework, five minutes of visualization before retiring and on awakening in the morning. It seemed a simple enough task for anybody wanting to get well.

"What should I think of?" he asked.

"Anything," said Dawn, "which shows your arm moving freely and perfectly."

Greg showed surprising apathy.

At the next session, four days later, Dawn asked, "Have you been programming your arm?"

He slumped into his seat. "I start to, but I fall asleep in the middle."

"How about in the morning?"

"I have to rush off to school."

She had finished hooking up the three machines, the EEG, the EMG, and the thermistor.

"You should work at it, Greg," she said, "as it should speed up the healing process."

"I'll try," he said perfunctorily. He looked curiously at the temperature device, registering 92 degrees.

"Try," she said, "to get the blood flowing to your hand."

The Alpha lights had flashed on brilliantly.

"What were you thinking?" she asked.

"I was moving my arm, and I saw the calcium deposits melting away."

"Don't put any calcium there; that's negative. Think of your arm as perfect and working perfectly at all times. Visualize it as lean, firm, sinewy, and in harmony with the rest of you, which is also perfect."

Greg nodded and closed his eyes.

The lights went on, and the EMG needle leaped forward, indicating a sharp muscle response.

"Did you move your arm?" she asked.

"No, I was just pushing Newcombe around the court again."

Dawn was concerned that the thermistor showed no activity, remaining at 92 degrees.

"Concentrate on warming your hand," she said.

"I've been visualizing it in a fire."

"That wouldn't do it," she said. "A burn suggests pain more than warmth."

"Well, I tried soaking it in a tub."

"Do you have a girl friend?" I put in.

He smiled slowly.

"Imagine yourself on a date in the moonlight."

"The moonlight went out with the fox trot."

He had taken his left hand, wired to the thermistor, and was rubbing it against his body.

"That won't do," said Dawn. "The impulse must begin in your head."

He kept the Alpha lights on and had the EMG needle moving. But he didn't seem able to work all three machines at the same time.

"It takes a little training," Dawn said. "Perhaps I should just connect him to the thermistor, so he can give it his full attention."

He closed his eyes and sat perfectly still. The thermistor needle made a few tentative movements. They were slight, but they were movements, the first since he had been hooked up to this machine.

"What were you thinking about?" Dawn quickly asked.

"I was lying on the beach, and the sun was streaming down, giving me a tan."

"Well, concentrate on that tan, and we'll see how quickly you improve."

She had been looking at his elbow. "Can you raise your arm over your head?"

He nodded and held his arm up.

"Can you move it to the side?"

He moved it easily.

"I can't quite straighten it out," he said. His extended fingers still couldn't touch his shoulder.

Dawn suggested he place his left hand over his right wrist and clasp it firmly as he tried turning the wrist first to the right and then the left. It was an old isometric exercise.

"This simple exercise may help you with your visualization. As you try to turn your wrist against the resistance of the other hand, see your elbow as strong and straight, in perfect harmony with your arm and the rest of the body. Do this at night, before retiring, and in the morning, and whenever you can during the day."

At no time, Dawn stressed, was Greg being exposed to psychotherapy. "If we can't help him with Biofeedback, then we're just not able to help him."

After a few sessions, Greg began to acknowledge some improvement. "My arm is getting better," he insisted. "I played some volleyball, which I hadn't done for a while, and it only hurt me for one day. Usually it would pain for four days."

Dawn smiled appreciatively and hooked up Greg to the EMG alone.

The needle, which had fluctuated widely during previous sessions, seemed stabilized below the five-microvolt mark.

"That's very encouraging," she said. "There's not as much activity in the elbow area."

"And what does that mean?"

"The circulation has subsided, indicating that the healing process has stabilized with the arm's improvement. You may recall that the needle jumped to forty-five microvolts at first."

Greg nodded serenely. "I guess I just know how to do it."

Dawn laughed. "If you're not careful, you'll release the arm completely, and then you'll be totally recovered."

"I want to get well," he protested.

Even so, he hadn't been doing the simple isometric exercise with the suggested visualization.

"I did it once," he said, "but it hurts."

"Think of it as being perfect," she said.

He looked up. "But pain is imperfection."

Dawn and I exchanged glances.

"Where did that idea come from?" Dawn asked gently.

He frowned. "The doctors said you shouldn't go through the threshold of pain."

Just at this point John Balog had poked his head into the Biofeedback room.

He smiled slightly and turned to Greg. "When a muscle hasn't been used for a while, there is bound to be some discomfort when you begin using it again. That doesn't mean you should overextend yourself or not be careful. Pain is not only a warning signal but a signal that your muscles are responding to the unaccustomed strain. You have to strike a balance, and you are the best judge of what that balance is."

It was a hot day, ninety degrees in the shade, and so I was scarcely surprised to see the thermistor needle move up a fraction.

As usual, Dawn asked what he had been thinking.

"How hot and uncomfortable it is."

As he stared, the needle moved again.

"What was it this time?" said Dawn.

"I just kept looking at it, telling it to move."

She laughed. "You should have told it to move up. It moved down.

In either case, though it indicated a certain conscious effort, it showed that the circulation to the elbow was being affected.

I had come across an article about a former Notre Dame football coach waging a successful fight against cancer. The doctors had given Joe Kuharich two years, and now, four years later, he was well enough to be talking about coaching again. He had refused to accept the medical verdict. "The doctors," he said, "based everything on biological and scientific reasoning. They left no margin for the will to live."

Dawn had the same cutting from a Pasadena newspaper.

"How come"—Greg turned to me suspiciously—"that you read a Pasadena newspaper?"

"I'm not trying to brainwash you," I said. "I saw it in a Los Angeles paper."

He slouched down in his chair and lazily stretched his legs. "It's fun to be sick," he said.

Dawn jumped at him. "Don't be negative."

He yawned. "I was only kidding."

"The thought is still framed in your mind."

"I still have calcium."

"Your arm should be perfect in your mind."

Greg showed a renewed interest as the temperature needle moved again.

"What are you thinking?"

"I'm in a sauna."

Machine-wise, Greg appeared to be progressing. After

several sessions, his EMG response was that of a normally healed arm, under five degrees when quiescent, yet still responsive to visual impulses. He could maintain Alpha at will, and was even beginning to show signs of controlling his circulation.

But he still complained of acute pain, spoke of calcium deposits, and was afraid to exercise normally lest he cause irreparable damage.

I had found myself liking the boy and involving myself in his recovery. And he appeared to respond to my interest. Perhaps that was the problem.

Dawn had suggested I stay on, and she was now regarding me speculatively.

"That injured elbow," I said, "may represent some advantage he doesn't want to give up."

"He should be further ahead," she acknowledged, "and he will be. But right now he is thinking more about what you want than what he wants." She paused a moment. "Normally there isn't an observer, and the subject feels secure in expressing whatever is on his mind."

I was inclined to agree. "I don't mind losing this trip twice a week."

And so the project went on without me.

In the third week, I received a call from Dawn. There was a happy edge to her voice. "Greg will be coming in for the last time tomorrow, and he'd like you to be here."

I hesitated a moment. "Is he ready to play tennis?"

"Come in," she said, "and meet the new Greg Porter."

Greg was already hooked up to the temperature sensor when I arrived. He seemed outwardly relaxed and had his customary smile. But, somehow, he looked different. His face seemed composed, and he no longer appeared a callow sixteen.

"You look mature," I decided.

He laughed. "I had a haircut."

"You look mature enough for tennis."

Dawn smiled. "Greg has made great progress, and he realizes he is better now. He has worked out a program for himself, which he wants to tell you about."

I looked at him inquiringly.

His eyes fell for a moment, then he looked at me evenly.

"My arm is well," he said with a trace of uncertainty, "but I don't think it's well enough for strenuous exercise as yet. I want to begin slowly, with swimming first and volleyball, continuing with basketball, then I'll eventually get into tennis." He gave his slow smile. "And I'll really drub you."

My face must have dropped, for I had equated his recovery with his taking to the courts and exerting his elbow with his former vigor.

"This is a big step forward," said Dawn. "Greg is making his own decision about himself for the first time. He thought it all out, and he knows exactly what is best for himself."

She gave me a cheerful look. "In a sense, this new confidence is the most beneficial thing that could have happened to him, and it should color his every activity from now on."

I said with a heartiness I didn't feel, "Well, if you're satisfied, and Greg is satisfied . . ."

I shook Greg's hand. "Come down and swim at my place. We have a big pool, all the way to Japan."

"Scuba diving," he said, "that's what I'll do."

Dawn beamed. "You see, he's telling you what he'll do."

After Greg left, Dawn and I faced each other across a battery of Biofeedback machines.

"He still isn't up to tennis," I said.

She laughed good-naturedly. "That's your criterion of success, and he has his own. You've seen the difference in him."

"He still seems to be blocking."

"Perhaps, but he has the equipment to work that out for himself now. He has the assurance that comes with deep relaxation, knowing that he can control his body and contact his inner mind at will."

I still had my doubts.

"How were all these wonders accomplished? Did he ever get the temperature sensor working?"

"He was able to raise it three degrees, displaying an impressive control over his own circulation."

"And how did he do that?"

"Just by relaxing, feeling his hand growing heavy and

199

warmer, while he thought about being in a sauna or on the beach."

"Did he do his homework?"

"He began visualizing five minutes, morning and night, thinking of whatever would help move his arm and increase its circulation. It came easier after he made the temperature sensor rise. He knew something was going on, and he was doing it."

But it hadn't been all that simple. Even when the machines were doing his bidding, Greg still complained that his arm pained him.

"What's wrong with the machine?" he had asked as the EMG indicated his arm was normal.

"Nothing," Dawn had said. "That machine is reflecting you."

"That may be, but it still hurts."

"Think about what that machine is telling you."

He had closed his eyes and thought.

"That my arm is well."

"Precisely. The pain is an old pattern that you're still clinging to. It's not truly you, or the machine would not reflect the increased muscle response of continued healing."

And so Greg, almost reluctantly, admitted that he must be well, for we live in a machine age that tells us machines don't lie.

"Once he was fully aware of the changes in himself— and the machine made that apparent—he was able to connect his performance to his own improvement."

"Will he continue to make progress?" I asked.

"I think so, because the change is within him."

"And what was the critical change?"

She smiled. "His deciding that he didn't need an excuse not to play tennis."

"Such as a bad elbow?"

Being a scientist, she wouldn't commit herself.

"Perhaps."

Chapter 18

A New World

"Greg Porter's mother would like to thank you for what you did," my secretary reported.

"I'm not sure he's that much better."

"Oh, it's not his arm," she laughed. "It's his personality. She says he's a changed person."

"In what way?"

"Oh, I don't know. Why don't you talk to her?"

Martha Porter was very specific. "I don't know what you people have been doing," she said, "but Greg has certainly improved. He's so considerate, I can hardly believe it. He used to tease his younger brother terribly, and now he's so solicitous."

The brother had hurt his wrist, and Greg, with unusual concern, had helped him into the house and given him first aid.

He had called from school once, and asked, "Are you all right, Mother? Is there anything I can do?"

Above all, she had sensed a more relaxed attitude, a new self-confidence, an absence of concern for himself and his own physical being.

I reported the apparent change to Dawn Balog. She was delighted. "As he keeps reaching new levels of thought," she said, "he is bound to become healthier in every way."

"The new Greg Porter," I said.

"Well, there wasn't that much wrong with the old Greg Porter. He just had to come into contact with his own mind and body, and that's what Biofeedback meditation has been doing for him."

Nobody expected Greg Porter to go through life with

electrodes attached to his head. But if his arm improved noticeably, as it had, and he resumed exercise, as he did, and if his sense of awareness about himself continued to mount, then it could be safely said that he was making use of his Alpha-Theta brainwaves.

Where it failed it was usually because the person had not made visual meditation an ongoing part of his life. As Dr. Balog had pointed out, it was often simpler to cling to advantages when what was to be gained didn't seem to compensate for what could be lost.

Even more important than getting well, perhaps, was staying well. And this could very easily be one of Alpha-thinking's major contributions. By relaxing at will, Balog felt, people could deliberately maintain their physical and mental well-being, bolstering their resistance against infection by heightening the immunity factor.

"Good heath is so often good thinking."

Student after student told me what Alpha-training had done for him on a continuing basis. "It's me," said eighteen-year-old Lisa Romary of the San Fernando Valley. "I'm not as nervous, understand my parents' problems, and what they expect of me. And yet I retain my individuality, in school and at home, and know that only I have the power to make the decisions affecting my life."

Kathy Marquardt of Milwaukee found the doorway to inner space. "I was living in the foyer of my apartment and didn't know it. Now with the door opened on the rest of my apartment, I realize that life is a unity and I am part of that unity, given a sense of universal goodness and direction that makes me want to flow with the tide of this goodness."

With the assurance born of self-mastery, she had discovered the ability to express affection and to stand up for the rights she had let slip away before, never too sure she had any. But it would have all ended in Bill Schwartz's classroom had she not continued to apply herself. It was something that had to be practiced every day, if only for a few minutes. "I now have the tools, for the first time, not only to understand my choice but to act on it."

With practice, many simplified getting into their levels. One businessman pulled on his ear lobe. Another used the finger and thumb technique. Still others just closed their eyes and were there.

"After a while," a graduate explained, "you establish a subconscious pattern, and this reduces the programming to one button instead of a series of buttons. The brain is capable of doing it all instantaneously."

He put every problem in pictures. "If I can see it, I know I can do it. Often I visualize the outcome, then start backtracking to the means. I don't understand how the intuitive mind works, any more than I know how electricity works, but I'm ready to profit by it. Some people won't accept an effect because they can't see the cause, and so close off their own growth."

My mind had gone back many times to San Rafael and the young mother with the azure blue eyes. I wondered not only what had happened to her but to her hapless daughter.

And then, one day, as if in answer to my unspoken message, she called.

She was as beautiful as ever. Neither time nor trouble seemed capable of touching her.

"What is your secret?" I asked.

She smiled. "In my meditation, I put my problems in the hands of one greater than I."

Again I was amazed by the freshness of her complexion and features. She seemed hardly more than a teen-ager herself.

She rested her chin in her hand for a moment. "I couldn't bear looking at that situation in the black frame of the Screen of the Mind, seeing it in its tragic seaminess, so I kept putting a white light around her and projected the courage for her to make a break."

I studied her for a moment. "Why didn't you put a light around him?"

"I did, every day, focusing on both of them. Separate pictures, of course, as I didn't want to suggest a continuing relationship."

On the day the daughter finally left her disturbed young man, instead of reacting violently, he behaved with a generosity he had never shown before.

"And where is she now?"

"She's home with me, where I visualized her, with a new friend."

"And did you visualize that, too?"

"Oh, yes, I knew she needed somebody, and so I programmed a young man who would be kind, intelligent, and loyal." She looked up at me. "And he looks just as I pictured him."

With most meditation, I noticed a new upswing in the spiritual, taking a priority over material concerns, even with very real material problems.

Spirituality was not a profession of sectarianism but of unity—within one's self, and with Creation. It was essentially good, not bad; optimistic, not pessimistic; involved, not detached. It was a swathe of life, as broad as the spirit itself.

"All through life," said Anne Francis, "people are programmed to feel guilty, until they have a very poor opinion of themselves." Like Carol Lawson, she had discovered that as you look at yourself candidly in your levels, you are never quite as bad as you thought.

"'Am I ready to accept my goodness?' That is the question you have to ask. Once a person meditates and is in contact with a power he can control, he frees himself of externally imposed strictures. He is in touch with the universe, and is spiritually on his way."

This new way was reflected in almost everything the actress did. "We were doing a lifeboat scene in a tank, and were constantly being pitched into the cold water. Instead of thinking how wet, cold, and bedraggled I was, I thought of the water as fresh, reviving, and warm, of the same infinite force as myself. And soon I felt warm and snug."

There were other occasions. "We were on location in the hills, and the rain was coming down in buckets. I looked at the sky and thought how magnificent it was, and how the weather was created by the same Creation that created me, and I felt at one with the whole scene, not only comfortable but exhilarated."

She smiled. "I was the only one who didn't catch cold."

I knew what Anne was saying. One day, I was strolling the beach with my dogs when the surf rolled in unexpectedly and drenched me to my knees. A cold wind blew up, and the wet trousers clung clammily to my legs and my feet squished around in salt water. I could remember when I would have nervously ended the walk and turned homeward, to slip off the sopping clothing and take a hot bath. And the next day, I would be down with a cold. This day, however, I continued on for another three or four miles, telling myself that my feet would get warmer as I kept on and that I would return refreshed and invigorated. And that was exactly how it worked out.

I still got an occasional headache, tensing over the typewriter in the early hours of the morning, but thought myself out of it, shunning the painkillers so universally popular. I strove for self-mastery, without which everything is our master. This didn't mean that I didn't go to a dentist when a tooth broke, or to an ophthalmologist when I needed glasses. It meant only that I myself decided what was best for me.

Alpha graduates were constantly prodded to prove their prowess.

"With all this awareness," some scoffed, "why not go to Las Vegas and make a bundle?"

Some had tried in a lighthearted way.

Linda Lockwood, now Bass, visiting a compulsive gambler in the Nevada resort, made seven passes in a row at the dice table. "I just knew I was going to seven, and told my friend. But he was intent on losing his own way, as compulsive gamblers do."

With this conviction, why hadn't she doubled up her bets?

"It was just fun," she said, "and I didn't want it to be anything else."

At the same resort, Michael Ellard spotted an elderly lady rolling the dice and betting a dollar. He tuned into a winning vibration and bet with her as she made sixteen straight points, an almost unbelievable mark.

"By the time her streak broke off," he said, "I couldn't carry my chips."

Why isn't everybody doing it?

"The desire for gain," observed teacher Pat Patrick, "is one of the most conscious of all motivations, and when people gamble purely to win, their conscious Beta minds will most likely block out the subconscious channel through which these hunches come."

In my research, I had shunned the academicians, the armchair generals who vied for the approval of their peers. I was impressed by the pragmatism of a Dr. Balog, motivated to help the sick, and by a Dr. William McGarey of Phoenix, Arizona, concerned more with enlightenment than scientific standards.

"Clinical research," said McGarey, "need not be a large activity—rather it is more important that things be done in decency and order, and that the truth be demonstrated, no matter if it is a single case."

With this outlook, he discussed the role of music therapy on the unconscious mind. "We are all familiar with the manner in which one type of music soothes us to sleep while another stirs our martial instincts. In Europe, the works of the masters are being played through a device that influences cell tissue by transforming sounds into direct vibrations. A Rome physician has been using Bach fugues to treat indigestion, and Mozart appears to be an ideal choice when working with rheumatism. Beethoven is considered good for hernias, while Handel helps 'broken hearts' and other disturbed emotional states."

For insomnia?—Schubert.

There were many experiments of the kind McGarey advocated. In Milwaukee, Dr. Winston W. Hollister, a physician, and his wife, Carol, a biologist, decided to test the physiological effects of meditation in a decent and orderly way.

One evening, after a particularly stressful day, including a talk before an assembly of physicians, Dr. Hollister decided to test the effect of meditation on blood pressure—his own.

"We got out the blood pressure cuff and stethoscope," said Carol, "and took his initial blood pressure: 126 over 98. This would have been low for some people, but was unusually high for my husband. He was concerned, and eager to see if meditation could bring it down."

They laid out very simple ground rules, since they were not trying to impress anybody but merely establish the truth. "We agreed that after five minutes, and again ten minutes of meditation, I would take blood pressure readings while he remained in a meditative state. The results were as follows:

"Five minutes: 116 over 86."

"Ten minutes: 110 over 78."

The systolic pressure, keyed to the heart's contraction, had decreased sixteen degrees, the diastolic, as the heart relaxed, was lower by twenty.

It was a classic example of self-mastery.

"During the meditation, Win actively thought about controlling his blood pressure, directing his body to relax, and telling himself that his blood pressure would decrease."

The conclusion was obvious.

"This simple experiment seemed to demonstrate the value of knowing how to control and direct your body, of having the ability to control body tensions due to stressful situations."

Why was it of supreme importance to immediately counter negative thinking on a positive level?

"If not turned aside," Dawn Balog observed, "these suggestions can very well be implanted in the subconscious mind, which is the seat of the memory, and negatively program mind and body."

The subconscious mind, reflected in Alpha-Theta thinking, remembered everything from a conscious level.

"It is reasonable to assume," said Dawn, "that as the subconscious mind opens up it eventually becomes more susceptible to suggestions on a conscious level."

The more sensitive the person, the more vulnerable he was. I recalled from newspaper days the prank played on the office hypochondriac, an extremely nervous type with a vivid imagination. As the victim came in and sat down at his desk, a colleague sauntered over leisurely, engaged him in idle conversation, then said with an air of concern, "What's wrong? You look a little pale."

"I do?" He put his hands to his face with a look of instant alarm.

A half hour passed, and then a second co-worker approached. He allowed a gleam of solicitude to appear in his eyes, without saying anything.

"What's wrong?" said the sensitized victim, leaping for the bait.

"Oh, it's nothing." The other shrugged.

The victim shot to his feet. "Please tell me what it is," he implored.

"Oh, just a look around the eyes. Nothing, really."

The city room watched gleefully as their impressionable colleague headed for the nearest mirror. When he returned minutes later, he looked pale and distraught.

He approached the city desk, with a hand on his forehead, and said in a tremulous voice:

"I have to leave. I have a fever."

The city editor gave him a withering look. "Sit down, you bum," he bellowed, to the delight of the city room. "You're sick in the head."

As gales of laughter broke out on all sides, the victim collapsed in his seat and managed somehow to get through the day.

The next day, he called in sick. And, as I look back, I am sure he was.

Hopefully, the time was ripe when physicians, generally, would make use of the positive aspects of the impressionable mind. A handful of pioneers were showing the way. Dr. Carl Simonton, a youthful Fort Worth radiologist, had taken Alexander's class and promptly started using what he had learned. His first patient was a former paladin of the Mafia, with terminal cancer of the throat. "He could scarcely breathe when I first saw him. He could not swallow, and could eat nothing. But he had an enormous will to live. I would tell him to do something three times a day, and he would do it five."

Simonton was criticized for prolonging the man's agony. But the patient responded and began to attack lesser ailments, using meditation on his arthritis. "He was also impotent and had had no sexual intercourse for twenty years. He got over this as well, had intercourse with his wife as often as they wanted, and jested he was ready to hire out as a stud."

At a California Air Force base, Simonton applied his techniques to severe cancer cases. On color slides, before an intrigued audience, the doctor picked out an ugly sore. The patient was a thirty-eight-year-old navigator. "This is a large cancer on his hard palate—he also had a cancer in

208

his throat. Everyone had pretty much given up hope. But he didn't buy that."

Successive slides showed the diminution of the ulcerated area. After six weeks, all signs of cancer had disappeared. Conventional therapy, which had been ineffective, had been continued. Additionally the patient had visualized himself as being well.

The more positive the attitude, the greater the response. "Negative-minded patients showed little or no response. With the less negative response, results were a little better. With intermediate attitudes, there were intermediate responses. And with fully cooperative, enthusiastic patients, doubly positive results."

He had drawn up a table showing the varying responses.

"Did they have hangnails?" the commanding general asked.

Colleagues asked why he used therapeutic machines when he was so high on his meditation techniques.

"Because I'm not smart enough yet," he replied.

He grew smarter with each patient. A pregnant woman had turned up with cervical cancer, and then an infection developed after the delivery. Traditional cancer treatment was delayed, and yet two weeks later her condition had improved. Everything in his experience told Simonton the woman should have gotten worse.

When he began treating her cancer, he explained that she was to visualize how her body consumed its own disease, thinking this three times a day.

She looked at him curiously. "That sounds like meditation."

"Did you meditate on your disease?" Simonton asked.

She nodded. "Yes, I did."

He regarded her with mounting excitement. "Do you think this had anything to do with your getting better?"

"Yes, I do."

He would have liked to use the meditation technique exclusively, but the risks were too great. "Hers was a very curable disease by standard methods. If for any reason we had failed, we would have been guilty of malpractice."

In the midst of miracles, I had my misgivings. If a Carolyn Carroll could program a mole off her mother's chest, why couldn't a contrary thought form a similar mole? In their enthusiasm, neophytes spoke in superlatives of Alpha's wonders, forgetting that an amateur diagnosis could be dangerous. Nor did they apparently fear the wide-ranging mental malpractice, the transmitting of evil, as dramatized in native voodoo.

The Alpha student, supporters maintained, was in a superior position to ward off negative programming by the very self-control he had secured for himself. "Where you have gained control of your own mind," observed Gael Pavek, a youthful Santa Monica schoolteacher, "your subconscious mind is automatically alerted to negative influences. You don't even have to think of them consciously. Your inner mind turns them off intuitively, whether it's a friend, the radio, television, or the newspapers."

She seemed so sure of herself that I couldn't help asking:

"Suppose somebody with Alpha-Theta powers put you on his Screen of the Mind in a black frame and projected your failure in all things?"

Gael's pretty face brightened. "But I wouldn't let him. In my levels, with my self-image on the Screen, I tell myself every day that this will be the most productive twenty-four hours of my life. I will do only good and have only good done to me." Her fair brow ruffled for a moment. "Actually there is more likelihood of somebody unfamiliar with Alpha-thinking beaming negative thoughts your way. For with Alpha, as a person becomes in tune with the universe, he tends to grow spiritually and is more concerned with helping his fellow man."

"Why this sudden concern for others?"

"We are all part of the same universe, and our lives are all interwoven. So as we help the totality of man, we are helping ourselves and those we love."

It seemed almost elementary, the way she put it.

"I've had my problems," she said, "and that got me into Pat Patrick's course."

"Did somebody psych you out?"

"Generally we make our own problems, in not knowing how to handle something. In my case, it was my own psychic experiences. They threw me into a panic."

Another student had reported she was quite psychic,

having correctly predicted a number of events in her future.

"There's nothing terribly traumatic about predicting," I observed. "You could always be wrong."

"Oh, it wasn't that. I would be lying down and see myself leaving my own body. I could see the mind part of me overhead, as if in space, and my body stretched out. I didn't know what it was, and the disassociation of mind and body was scary."

"That happens frequently in meditation," I said.

She smiled rather grimly. "Yes, but I didn't know that then."

She went to professional psychics looking for an explanation, and then decided to learn the Alpha technique, not only to develop but to master her burgeoning powers. In the process, she had now achieved a certain self-mastery. "Your inner level recognizes the truth and responds only to that truth."

"And truth is goodness?"

"Exactly. And so let all the demons do their worst. They can't do a thing, particularly when we know that the worst demon is the one within ourselves."

Elmer Green, fearful of clumsy teaching techniques that breed "demons," had posted his guidelines for an ideal mind-training program.

"Permit each person to discover himself at a proper rate, penetrating the unconscious [mind] at a rate consistent with his ability to keep his feet on the ground. Those for whom psychic unfoldment would lead to destructive neuroses should obtain only those insights which would help integrate and control various discordant sections of the personality.

"The student should be shielded from teacher imperfections that might otherwise become part of the student's psychic atmosphere.

"Teachers should be evaluated according to their awareness, so that as each student progresses he has a properly qualified *human* adviser [none of those assistants].

"Training centers for self-awareness should be within access of anyone interested, on a nonprofit basis."

My own feeling, like Balog's was that Alpha-training should be incorporated in the schools, taught by qualified people, but not necessarily people with degrees, who responded to students at their level of need.

I had heard scattered reports of students suffering bad experiences but, in talking to literally thousands, had never encountered anything like it. However, I sympathized with Dr. Green's concern. I recalled the brashness of one greedy teacher, looking over his class of twenty, each paying two hundred dollars for the privilege of his teaching, and saying:

"This is hardly worth my while."

As I had learned from Alexander, so had I passed on his course in the hope that others could profit without a teacher if none was available.

By following the inductive exercises set down by Alexander, repeating the color, countdown and passive nature visualizations as we did in class, it is only a matter of time before the reader schools himself into the mind state of the classroom student. He can readily create his own Workshop, visualize his own Screen and dramatize the events and changes he wishes to achieve. He may heighten the subconscious by communing with the four seasons and visualizing himself in an expanding block-house of lead, or reduce a migraine headache, stop smoking, lose weight or end insomnia with Alexander's specific techniques. If reading silently or aloud is not effective, perhaps the reader can tape the material and play it back. That should do it, if nothing else does.

I saw no more of Cathy Francis, who had gotten me into it all, but learned that she had married. I somehow felt that, like Linda Lockwood, she had visualized her husband as she needed him and he had appeared. I was sure it would be that simple for her.

Alexander, meanwhile, in San Francisco, had developed a new course, "Samata," symbolizing the balance which is the road to successful living. "You will learn," he told students, "about the fourfold nature of man—physical, emotional, mental, spiritual—and how to bring the four levels into one harmonious whole."

I would hardly have recognized him after all these years.

His hair was long and a little unruly, and he sported an open shirt and slacks. A chain dangled from his neck, with a symbol of man's fourfold nature. But the principal changes, as with Ernie Dade, appeared more than skin-deep. This was a humbled Alexander, with a clear eye and a quick smile. He was able to jest about his lack of humor, showing a surprising humor.

"What happened?" I asked.

"I've mellowed."

It was more than that, and we both knew it.

"Perhaps," said Alexander, "I've learned from my students. You know, teaching can be a two-way process."

Alexander, I decided, was no longer the stuffy English schoolmaster, but a universal man born of the mind experience he had shown so many. He was, happily, not unique. Wherever one went, people were newly concerned with enriching their lives. There was growing discontent with static roles that programmed dullness and dreariness, even with the sop of security, from cradle to grave. There was a yearning to know more about one's place in the universe, to commune realistically with the order we dimly perceive about us in the stately procession of the planets and the predictable cycles of the seasons. For the first time, man had a tool to probe the mystery of his own existence, with intuitive flights of insight capable of revamping the whole desultory scheme of imitative education. In knowing himself, he would know also the world he lived in.

The human spirit was rising with new force to meet the challenge of a worldly ennui and defeatism. It was never too late for anybody who didn't find it too late. A retired businessman talks about his life having slipped away, then asks hesitatingly:

"Can this new awareness, this new mind-training, help us understand who we are?"

"Hopefully, it is a beginning."

"Does one have to be religious?"

"People work it into their own background. It is fundamentally a technique to learn about ourselves."

I remembered the message of a young psychiatrist, Dr. Robert Constas:

"It is indeed possible to continue growing, in wisdom and inner power, beyond the age of twenty-one. There is an inner Healer within each of us which can be experi-

213

enced as a beauty and love, a wisdom and a power, an active liberating force."

With meditation and visualization, the inner Healer can be released so that vitalizing energy can flow through the individual and keep him wonderfully well and productive. This Healer is the inner self, the subconscious thought, the new awareness, the Alpha-Theta, the new dimension of the mind, the point of contact at which the individual sees his true self in the mirror of the world about him. And it is all out there, waiting. For as was said two thousand years ago:

"And I say unto you, Ask, and it shall be given you; seek, and ye shall find; knock, and it shall be opened unto you."

Appendix

Do-It-Yourself Exercise to Alpha

For the convenience of the reader who plans a do-it-yourself program the steps to Alpha-thinking are here reviewed:

Settle yourself comfortably, and take a deep breath, allowing the mind to drift leisurely. Relax the shoulders and neck, and, hopefully, the rest of the body will take a hint. Your conscious mind may be restless at first, but don't let that bother you. It is normal. Begin your first countdown, thinking of each numeral as a step. Always visualize, whatever the specific exercise. On the countdown from twenty-one, which can be ticked off silently or aloud, drift deeper and deeper with each number into the very core of your being. See that core as something substantial, however it comes to you.

On this countdown you may pause briefly at intervals of three, as student Linda Lockwood did, to scan your own muscles, skin, bones and nerves mentally. After reaching the count of one, continue to relax. At this deeper and more inward level, visually pick out a passive scene from nature that is meaningful to you, still keeping the eyes closed. Become calm, still, at peace, and see yourself within this scene from nature. Enjoy it. In my own case, I pictured the rolling waves breaking on the surf outside my Pacific window. Sit this way, eyes closed, body relaxed, for as long as you like, putting aside all conscious thinking as your imagination roams over this scene.

Again, take a deep breath, and still, with the eyes closed, move mentally through the colors of Alexander's rainbow. Each color should suggest a different and vivid sensation. As you continue to relax, getting ever more deeply into your subconscious levels, see first the color Red, visualizing an apple, if you will. See yourself biting into it. With the color Orange, visualize an orange, and consider the times you have been needlessly upset emotionally. Needlessly is the watchword. With Yellow, bask in the golden sunshine of your mind, and grow even calmer. With the soothing color Green, you visualize the forest and inner peace; with Blue, the azure sky and a feeling of love; with Purple, the mystical twilight; and, with Violet, a misty haze gradually merging into the endless sea. The student, if he feels more comfortable thereby, may run through the rainbow first and then go into the countdown, sandwiching the passive scene from nature between the two. In the beginning I found the countdown a more effective way of proceeding into my own levels.

Now mentally create a large screen some distance away. Make this screen as large as you like. Design it to your own tastes, for this is to be your Screen of the Mind. On this Screen of the Mind, which could resemble Cinerama's living color, visualize ten pictures in sequence, increasing your ability to visualize and imagine. Put a white light around the frame of what you see, and always visualize the problem or project in light.

You are now ready to visualize the elevator which will take you into your imaginary Workshop at the count of three. Or you can walk down, if you will, using twelve steps. Make the Workshop into what you want it to be visually. Preferably, it should be a large room, capable of containing everything you will require. In my own case, I installed a large oblong table, similar to the copydesk of a newspaper city room, a television set, a telephone, a walkie-talkie, chairs, tables and a comfortable couch for reclining. All these are optional and help stimulate your creative faculties.

Every Workshop has its raised platform and its Screen of the Mind at one end of the room. Whatever problems you wish to solve are projected like a motion picture onto the platform or the Screen of the Mind, where a radiant white light is put around them.

The student sits comfortably at his desk, which he

may take the count of twelve to get to, leisurely examining the furniture and decorations as he crosses the room to take his place. On either side of him, in equally comfortable chairs, he installs an imaginary assistant, whom he can pick deliberately, or who, at this point, may present himself through the now altered awareness of Alpha-thinking. Whenever in a quandary, the student can mentally turn to his assistants for help.

With practice, the beginner will find, as so many students have, that he can by-pass the preliminary stages —the rainbow and the count downs—and go directly to his Workshop and the Screen of the Mind.

Some have found that with the circle technique, forming a circle with thumb and index finger, they immediately slip into the problem-solving stage of Alpha. Others surround themselves with the white light associated with the Screen of the Mind and are able to help themselves and others.

After a while in visualizing the colors of the rainbow or the Screen of the Mind I could very quickly get into my Alpha levels. However, visualization had to be practiced daily or the facility slackened off and vanished. Sometimes meditation was difficult and the mind wandered restlessly. On one such occasion, drawing on the experience of others, I immersed myself in an infinity of white light which gave off a loving, restorative quality. As I concentrated on this light, which diffused itself into a glowing nimbus of a cloud, I began to associate with it an infinite, all-knowing intelligence. My whole being blended with this radiance, as I was made aware of this infinite presence, this inner healer, expressed as beauty and love, wisdom and power. I was conscious of a new liberating force and felt a sudden rise and flow of energy. I felt myself regaining a center of awareness, an identifying strength which intuitively told me the right course for myself. The counsel and advice of others seemed superficial, even superfluous. The answer, as for us all, lay within the deeper layers of the mind and in our relation to the universal force about us. I now understood what that young Vietnam veteran had meant when he said: "For the first time in my life I realize that I have a companion who is part of me just as I am part of him, somebody who loves me just as I love him."

And I, too, like everybody else, was part of that universe and had the same help. None of us was alone.

Index

JESS STEARN was born in Syracuse, New York. After studying at Syracuse University he embarked on an active career in journalism, writing for most of the major newspapers including the Hearst group, Scripps-Howard, and *Newsweek* magazine, with his series on schools, crime, narcotics, etc., winning him many awards. Most notably, the Front Page Award was presented to him by the American Newspaper Guild for his cover story on Joseph P. Kennedy.

His books in the psychic field have all been groundbreakers, helping get both scientific people and the general public interested in this area. His previous NAL books *Adventures Into the Psychic* and *A Time for Astrology* have received awards and praise from professional circles as well as having been best sellers.